HOMESTEADING

Mastery of Gardening With Business and Profitability Guide

(A Comprehensive Guide to Aquaponic Gardening)

Barbara Crawford

Published by Harry Barnes

Barbara Crawford

All Rights Reserved

Homesteading: Mastery of Gardening With Business and Profitability Guide (A Comprehensive Guide to Aquaponic Gardening)

ISBN 978-1-7778032-8-5

All rights reserved. No part of this guide may be reproduced in any form without permission in writing from the publisher except in the case of brief quotations embodied in critical articles or reviews.

Legal & Disclaimer

The information contained in this book is not designed to replace or take the place of any form of medicine or professional medical advice. The information in this book has been provided for educational and entertainment purposes only.

The information contained in this book has been compiled from sources deemed reliable, and it is accurate to the best of the Author's knowledge; however, the Author cannot guarantee its accuracy and validity and cannot be held liable for any errors or omissions. Changes are periodically made to this book. You must consult your doctor or get professional medical advice before using any of the suggested remedies, techniques, or information in this book.

Upon using the information contained in this book, you agree to hold harmless the Author from and against any damages, costs, and expenses, including any legal fees potentially resulting from the application of any of the information provided by this guide. This disclaimer applies to any damages or injury caused by the use and application, whether directly or indirectly, of any advice or information presented, whether for breach of contract, tort, negligence, personal injury, criminal intent, or under any other cause of action.

You agree to accept all risks of using the information presented inside this book. You need to consult a professional medical practitioner in order to ensure you are both able and healthy enough to participate in this program.

Table of Contents

INTRODUCTION 1

CHAPTER 1: ADVANTAGES OF HOMESTEAD FOOD PRODUCTION 13

CHAPTER 2: BUILDING TECHNIQUES 26

CHAPTER 3: BEST ANIMALS FOR HOMESTEADING 43

CHAPTER 4: HOW MUCH LAND 48

CHAPTER 5: HOMESTEAD LIFE HACK 67

CHAPTER 6: INTRODUCTION TO INDOOR GARDENING 72

CHAPTER 7: HOMESTEAD LIFE HACKS 76

CHAPTER 8: THE IMPORTANCE OF SEED SAVING 88

CHAPTER 9: MAINTAINING YOUR VEGETABLE GARDEN .. 91

CHAPTER 10: HOW TO MAKE A LIVING HOMESTEADING. 98

CHAPTER 11: BACKYARD HOMESTEADING 108

CHAPTER 12: VITAL EQUIPMENT FOR HOMESTEADERS . 114

CHAPTER 13: HOW TO PREPARE YOUR NUT AND FRUIT ORCHARD 120

CHAPTER 14: WAYS TO BECOME AN URBAN HOMESTEADER 153

CHAPTER 15: HOW TO CREATE AN AMAZING HOMESTEAD GARDEN 166

CHAPTER 16: HOMESTEAD IN THE HOME 180

CHAPTER 17: FAST GROWING VEGETABLES FOR A SPRING GARDEN 184

CONCLUSION 188

Introduction

Understanding Homesteading

In this relentless innovation-driven world, carrying on with life at a moderate and loosening up pace has begun to pick up ubiquity and acknowledgment. Rising expansion, overdependence on innovation, deficiency of assets, pesticides ridden foods grown from the ground, and not-a-second to-recover way of life have driven various individuals into taking a gander at homesteading as a suitable way of life. In spite of the fact that homesteading is surely not another idea, the thoughts and ideas of metropolitan homesteading have begun to pick up footing with both the youthful and the metropolitan populace.

Previously, homesteaders went through years undertaking backbreaking assignments of furrowing, plowing, and reaping ranches cut out of the complete wild. They avoided cutting edge pleasantries and devices. Albeit, present-day homesteaders too attempt genuinely thorough undertakings, they are, in any case, not as tiring as the past day assignments. However, let this not fool you as homesteading — present or past — is burdening in the event that you don't have the correct fitness to carry on with your existence without various supposed 'essential' pleasantries that we underestimate.

Countless individuals are pulled in towards homesteading in light of the fact that it helps keep unfortunate and destructive synthetic substances out of the evolved way of life. Going to cultivating is the best way to guarantee that all of us approach healthy and less-tainted food. Also, individuals have gone further and have guaranteed that synthetics don't discover their way into their own lives too. With each move they make, homesteaders ensure that they don't hurt themselves, their co-creatures, the Earth, and the people in the future. Call it what you may — green development, eco cognizant, or becoming environmentally friendly — the essential thought that characterizes homesteading is independence and natural obligation. Homesteading, as troublesome and backbreaking it may appear at first, is the initial move towards a more joyful, more beneficial, and fulfilling way of life.

Metropolitan homesteading is anything but another idea or thought; truth be told, homesteading is as old as the mountains. Before individuals began purchasing bread and eggs from stores, everybody brought poultry up in their terraces and prepared bread at their homes.

Homesteading is an old idea; nonetheless, metropolitan homesteading has resuscitated the old procedures of independence and adjusted them to suit the metropolitan occupants' needs. Metropolitan homesteading is definitely not a solitary idea; it is an assortment of different methods and practices. It incorporates developing vegetables and natural products, raising creatures, protecting food, making bread, cheddar and yogurt at home, turning and sewing, making cleaning items, utilizing sun based and wind vitality, moderating water, and making manure and fertilizer. The one idea that holds metropolitan and rustic homesteading is simply giving, opposing the compulsion to gorge utilization, expending items made at home, making items instead of buying mass-delivered items from stores.

In the event that you need to carry on with an independent life, homesteading is an unquestionable requirement for you. Homesteading is marked by resource cultivating, home protection of groceries and it might in specific occurrences include a minor creation of garments, textures, and craftwork for home use or deal.

Homesteading for the most part makes a qualification from the provincial collective business by disconnection, socially, or truly of the ranch. The utilization of this term, in the United States of America, dates route back to the Homestead Act of 1862 and likely even before the nineteenth century.

Independence developments in the 20thcentury started to utilize the idea to city and rural areas known as metropolitan homesteading. It consolidates little reasonable cultivating and homemaking. In homesteading, government and social help coordination are regularly given a wide billet to support confidence and friends and relatives' hardship, to augment independence and self-assurance.

The level of independence occurs along with a range, with a lot of homesteaders delivering staples or exchanges to interest very good quality specialty purchasers so as to cover money related prerequisites. A few homesteaders go into this way of life following productive vocations which make accessible the subsidizing for power, generators, land, ranch hardware, lodging, sunlight based boards, and expenses.

Contemporary government rules as structure codes, food government assistance programs, zoning rules, least pay, and federal retirement aide for occasional work power. Also, town council limits on finishing, and creature authority have improved the peripheral cost of home creation of food.

Joined with the late awards of framing a feasible cultivating site, this increments the difficulty of setting up an autonomous estate starting from the earliest stage, for those of pitiful salary. Real financial investment funds from executing a homesteading presence show up most emphatically identified with second rate material resource guidelines and upkeep of bought means, for example, staple, power, water, and manure instead of diminishing expenses of presence.

Economies of measure in present-day cultivating and opportunity cost of physical work repress home-raised food things from being a practical decision. Numerous homesteaders notwithstanding, show profound endorsement with their norm of presence and feel that their method of living is more beneficial and preferred remunerating over other traditional types of living.

The following is a halfway posting of homesteading capacities that ideally may rouse new homesteaders to examine. This is strongly prescribed for youngsters who need to set out finding another way to deal with life. Every ability that you secure will be a stage closer to the existence of better confidence and independence.

Crucial homesteading aptitudes comprise of figuring out how to:

Bake bread;

Butcher small livestock such as chicken and rabbits;

Caponize a chicken;

Choose a location for a vegetable garden or orchard;

Cook 10 basic meals from scratch on a cook stove;

Crochet;

Cut and glaze glass;

Determine an animal's age by its teeth;

Dig and properly use a shallow well;

Do basic sewing; and home canning and food preservation;

Dub a chicken;

Dye cloth or yarn from plants;

Entertain yourself and live without electronic media;

Fillet and clean a fish;
Graft baby animals onto a foster-mother;
Grind wheat into flour;
Grow a vegetable plant and everyday kitchen herbs;
Haggle like a horse trader;
Hand thresh and winnow oats, wheat and other small grains;
Hang clothes on a clothesline;
Hatch out chicken, duck or other poultry eggs;
Knit;
Know the contrasts among trees and the remarkable properties of different kinds of wood; how and when to utilize crossover seeds; how and when to prune grapes and organic product trees; when winter is finished; and solid plants and creatures from those which are not beneficial;
Lay fundamental block or fabricate a stone divider;
Realize when it is more efficient to purchase something instantly or when to make it yourself alongside fundamental pipes and how to perspire copper lines and joints;

Light a fire both inside and outside;
Live inside your money related methods;
Make hard or delicate cheddar; spread; wiener; paper and ink; candles; cleanser from wood remains and creature fat; fire starters from pinecones or corn cobs; make and utilize a hotbed or cold edge; and long haul plans for the future, for example, plan for a plantation or animals reproducing program;
Make your own wine;
Oversee human pee and excrement without plumbing;
Purify milk;
Plant a tree;
Appropriately utilize a handsaw, estimating tape; hammer and nails, wire cutters, and screwdriver;
Peruse the climate, a chronological registry, the moon, and the stars;
Perceive your own psychological and physical expertise limits;
Resurface furniture;
Reload ammo;
Securely utilize a cutting tool;
Spare open-pollinated seeds;

Put lure snares for undesirable vermin and predators;

Sew your own clothing;

Hone any edge device, for example, an etch, blade, scraper, or hatchet;

Turn fleece, flax, or cotton into yarn or string with a drop shaft or on a turning wheel;

Trade, organization, and deal with similar individuals;

Tell the hour of the day by the sun;

Defrost solidified lines without busting them;

Utilize a scraper, garden scoop or spade without harming your back, a washtub, washboard and hand wringer; non-electric lighting; a lever sewing machine; a grass shearer; a weight cooker; a wood oven and how to bank a fire; electric netting or fencing; and a weight tank garden sprayer, a drill and do fundamental cowhide fix;

Weave fabric and a container; and,

Witch for water with a curve metal holder or forked branch.

These abilities are nevertheless a couple of the first homesteading aptitudes that an individual ought to have. The attention in this is on metropolitan homesteading which alludes to a family that produces for utilization a huge bit of their food in the type of vegetables, foods grown from the ground.

This is ordinarily to interface with the longing of the family in the said family to live in a naturally cognizant manner. Metropolitan homesteading, likewise called diversion cultivating or terrace homesteading features:

Network exchanging;

Fertilizing the soil;

Line drying of garments;

Developing organic products, culinary plants, vegetables, and therapeutic plants;

Homes with gardens, not yards;

Creation and conservation of food and items for home use;

Water collecting and utilization;

Raising chickens, hares, worms, goats, fish or honey bees;

Independent way of life through re-utilizing, finishing and reusing things; and

Use of elective force sources and methods for transport.

Grow your own foods grown from the ground.

Raise livestock for food • Use elective wellsprings of vitality — sustainable power source • Rethink transportation by utilizing bikes or strolling to work • Make endeavors to lessen squander and furthermore repurpose squander • Rainwater harvesting • Do your housework yourself • Learn to knit, mend, do repairs and learn using basic tools and techniques

Make food at home such as cheese, bread and yogurt.

Chapter 1: Advantages Of Homestead Food Production

Social benefits
It can be done on small plots of land, both in rural and urban areas (even for people who don't own land) increases availability, accessibility and utilization of nutritious food, offering a supplement to staple foods on a continuous basis. Homestead gardening has the potential to decrease 'hidden hunger' can easily be combined with day-to-day domestic activities and employment patterns of women. Therefore it can contribute to the empowerment of women and the nutritional situation of women and children (increased consumption of fresh fruits and vegetables).

Economic benefits
Growing your own fruits and vegetables is less expensive than buying products on markets. In addition a share can be sold,

providing the household with livelihood opportunities and an additional source of income.

Environmental benefits

It delivers a range of ecosystem services, especially when ecological friendly approaches are used. This is often the case, since little external inputs are used. Gardens are often diverse, growing multiple crops and plants and indigenous species, hereby contributing to biodiversity and conservation of natural resources. Gardens can provide a habitat for animals and organisms, contribute to nutrient recycling, land conservation and fertility, a reduction of soil erosion and enhances pollination. The use of plant material as fodder for animals and animal manures as compost to fertilize plants reduces the needs for chemical fertilizers. Thereby, gardens can provide a source for kindling and alternative sources of fuel, manure, building materials and animal feed.

Increasing benefits of homestead food production

Introducing applied techniques and improve knowledge can make home stead food production more beneficial, efficient and effective. Areas and issues to focus on include:

Market appraisal: meeting market needs, transportation, develop marketing strategies and understanding demand and supply.

Storage possibilities: to increase 'shelf life' and cover needs during shortage period.

Selection of garden products: involve everyone in the household on what to grow to meet household needs and preferences within the boundaries of available resources.

Adding value: through storage and small scale processing: increasing the livelihood options for rural households.

Marketing: knowing the customer and the market and improve entrepreneurial skills.

Organizations: organize and plan the division of tasks, complexity of the garden and products.

Service and input availability/development: skills and techniques, seeds, cuttings and seedlings. Fertilizers and other inputs and equipment, packaging material, market information.

Cultural Practices of Homestead Garden

Farmers generally collect planting materials from homesteads wildings (species that are grown/collected from outside homestead premises), friends and families, relatives, government, and NGO nurseries. No specific spacing is followed in planting of species in homestead garden. Sometimes it was also found to plant herbaceous species like Zingiber officinale, Curcuma longa under the layer of shrub like Carica papaya, Citrus limon, and so forth in order to make the optimum use of their land.

Study figured out the analysis of respondents answers regarding different aspects of the existing management systems of homestead gardens in the study area. During survey, it was found that some households are not engaged in any management/cultural operations in their homestead gardens whereas other households are more or less engaged with the management of homestead gardens. Species were planted usually during the morning and/or afternoon of the day mostly in the monsoon season. Generally, fast growing and species having low crown coverage are selected for the plantation. The results revealed that almost all the households carried out watering (100%) and soil ploughing (94%). Weeding was done out by 85% of respondents as well as fencing (53.75%) and 67.5% respondents did mulching. Consequently about 62% respondents practice thinning or pruning in their homestead garden. Large farmers generally hired labour for doing thinning and pruning operations.

But they do very much little care for manuring (46.25%) and applying pesticide (35%) in their homestead.

Perceived Importance for Conservation of Homestead Garden Species

To determine the perceived importance of homestead species conservation, farmers were interviewed using a questionnaire;

asked to evaluate the importance of mentioned eight functions of trees. Likewise, farmers' perceived most importance for homestead plant species conservation was related to fruit and food (85%) followed by building materials (78.75%), subsistence family income (73.75%), and source of firewood (68.75%). The surveyed rural area is affected by monsoon flood every year; as a result soil erosion is a serious problem in this region. Therefore, in order to keep houses above the water level, it is mandatory to raise houses at the highest elevations or fill the land by soil in the dry season, especially throughout the floodplain regions. As a consequence, people are usually concerned about the trees role to protect their homestead land against water-induced soil erosion by binding the soil. However, they were not concerned about ecological importance of forest.

Yet the majority of the respondents graded the homestead garden as being "less important" as a means of maintaining ecological balance and soil erosion control (37.5%), followed by a source of medicinal plants (35%). So, it seems that there is still a lack of knowledge in these two categories, and institutional and government and NGOs training and learning programs are necessary to facilitate knowledge.

Homestead gardening: Growing What You Eat

You can start small by growing just one food item this year, or you can jump in and create an entire garden. Either way, here are a few things to think about in the planning stages:

Available space– How much available space you actually have will determine what you are able to grow, but don't be discouraged. With a little research, you may discover you can grow things in different ways than you'd imagined. Raised bed gardens, hanging baskets, container gardening all open up opportunities for planting.

Sunlight– Observing how much sun and shade your growing spaces get will also impact what you can grow. Monitor your space for sunlight and study how much sun the food you'd like to grow requires.

Soil– The essential aspect of successful growth is good soil. Make sure you know what type of soil you have and amend it to meet the needs of what you want to grow.

Surrounding Vegetation– Trees require a lot of water and nutrients, so make sure you plant your garden away from competing foliage.

Support– Tending vegetable and other edibles requires time and attention. Get your family on board to help out and make some great memories, too.

Natural Care for your Garden
Soil Care

You need to keep caring for your soil so it does not get depleted of nutrients or have issues with soil erosion. Here are some things to research and consider:

Make Your Own Compost: Compost is important for your garden soil. You can continually buy some, but that will get bothersome and expensive. Another option is to make your own compost (click here to instructions). This will not only boost your garden soil for free, it will reduce your garbage disposal, which helps the environment and possibly your wallet.

Vermiculture: Another option for composting is vermiculture, which uses worms to break down your trash items for your soil. I prefer doing both a compost pit outdoors and a small bin of vermiculture indoors, since it will add a complexity to my compost soil for my garden by adding the two types together. Research both types and do what works best for your garden.

Fertilizer: I really hope that you will avoid commercial fertilizer products whenever possible. I understand that sometimes certain plants or soils need extra care in the form of fertilizer. Please research all natural possibilities before grabbing those generic store-bought fertilizers. My absolute favorite natural fertilizer product is fish emulsion. Made from fish parts (duh), fish emulsion is high in nitrogen and other helpful nutrients for your soil. Make sure to buy a good-quality organic one (like this one).

Crop Rotation: Another way to keep your garden soil healthy and happy is with crop rotation. Various fruits and vegetables fall in different plant families. Each plant family is susceptible to certain pests and bacteria. If you keep planting your cucumbers in the same spot every year, that soil can become stressed, weak, and very poor. Careful crop rotation is actually beneficial to your garden because some plant families gets boosts from the stuff that other plant families leave behind.

Soil Protectors: One common issue with soil is erosion. Wind, weeds, and even the sun can damage the top layer of soil, leaving it in bad condition. Fortunately, there are many options to help keep your topsoil happy. One option for protecting your garden soil are weed cover fabrics (like this one). I personally prefer mulch. You can use many different items for mulching your soil: cardboard, newspapers, leaves, hay, or actual mulch.

It depends on what is the best price for your budget.

Mulch keeps your soil moist longer (which will keep your water bills down) and protect your soil from damage and weeds. Click here to learn more about deep mulching your garden.

Cover Crops: Most gardeners either take winter off from gardening, or have just a few winter crops still going strong. One of the best ways to protect the topsoil of your garden during the winter is by planting cover crops. Each type of cover crop will give your soil a boost of different nutrients, so you can plan on planting different cover crops in different parts of your garden (based on your crop rotation plan) or make sure to get a specific cover crop that will be good for all the plants you decide to grow in the next spring.

Water Care

Watering your garden can be expensive unless you plan things out right. Here are some ways you can water your garden without breaking the bank and also giving them the best watering possible:

Mulch: As stated above, mulching will help keep your plants moist longer, so you won't have to water as much.

Make Rain Barrels: Rain Barrels will collect rain water (these are great around your home/garage/barn to collect water from your gutters) so you are not spending as much money on water bills. Rain water is very good water for your plants, too, so it will make your plants extra happy. Here's a great tutorial on making a rain barrel.

Drip Irrigation: drip irrigation will help keep your plants evenly moist and will also prevent wasted water. It can be expensive at first, but well worth it in the end to do drip irrigation. Here's a book that might help you understand drip irrigation better.

Bugs

There is pretty much no way can you have a garden without interacting with bugs. Bees, earwigs, spiders, and anything else you can think of, bugs live in the garden.

Don't let that stop you from gardening. Here are some things to consider:

Make a Bug Hotel: Not all bugs in the garden are bad bugs! In fact, some bugs are very beneficial to your garden's health. It can be hard to encourage them to live in your garden, but if you give them a place to live, they might just stick around. Here's a great tutorial on how to build a bug hotel. These things are beautiful.

Encourage Pollinators: Most plants will not provide you with food until they have been visited by pollinating insects. One of the best ways to get more pollinating bugs to your garden is by planting certain plants in your garden to attract them. Here is a great list of things to plant to encourage pollinators.

Natural Care for the Gardener

Make a Gardener's Hand Cream to sooth your skin after a hard day in the garden. Make a homemade and natural bug repellent spray to keep bugs away from you while you work in the garden. Make a homemade salve for bug bites, in case the repellent spray did not keep all of the bugs away and you get bit.

Have an herbal poison ivy remedy ready to use, if you are susceptible to poison ivy.

Chapter 2: Building Techniques

When constructing you home, there are many methods to choose from. For homesteaders, standard construction methods and materials are often not an option. Either the nearest lumber yard is too far away, too expensive, or those materials are simply considered not "green" enough. The two most popular "green" methods today, are log homes and cob homes.

First, lets look at cob construction. Cob can be used to make efficient, safe, and durable homes. Unlike many other materials, cob can easily be made and repaired with materials found around the yard. Though it is recommended that you study some detailed instructions and building plans, the basic concept is quite simple. Cob is a mixture of 50-70% sand, 15-30% clay, and 10-40% straw. The spcific proportions will vary depending on the type of clay in your area. Therefore, it is recommended that you make a few small test batches to get the right mix. After thoroughly mixing the sand, clay and straw, add a small amount of water and begin kneading the mixture like dough. Generally, for larger amounts of cob, this is done by laying out the ingredients on a tarp and kneading with your feet. Similar to stomping grapes for wine. Continue kneading and adding small amounts of water until the mixture is able to hold its shape when rolled into a ball or cylinder. While still wet, begin stacking, forming and shaping your house, shed, or other building project. The forming process is similar to clay sculpting. Generally, for ease of labor, the cob will be formed into large "bricks" which are then stacked together. Those bricks can then be shaped and molded, and will bond together as they dry. When the mixture dries it produces a material similar to cement, though not quite as hard. To prevent errosion from rain, the surface can be "painted" with natural oils such as linseed oil.

The designs you can build range from basic to quite artistic. The ability to form and shape the cob freely, allows you to use many designs that would be impossible with other materials. Cob is also a good material for constructing a wood stove and oven. Many cob homes incorporate a large round wood stove made of cob right in the center of the home. Some designs also include a small loft space with the floor of the loft being an extension from the body of the stove. This space is then used as a bedroom. The cob floor is warmed by the stove but will not get hot and makes for quite a cozy sleeping area.

One word of caution, when building a cob floor, it is highly recommended that you first build the floor out of timbers and then use layers of cob on top of those timbers. The timbers will give your floor extra strength, and in the case of a ground level floor, the timbers will keep the cob out of the moisture which will make it last longer. Done properly, a cob home can outlast more modern construction methods significantly. There are many cob homes today in the UK and other parts of Europe, that are more than 100 years old.

As for log homes, the designs are generally fairly simple, but with enough time and labor they can be quite lavish. There are a variety of methods for actually assembling a log home, but the traditional method is to use notches to lock the logs together. This is exactly the same method used in the classic Lincoln Logs toys, just on a different scale. Though your timbers don't need to be completely squared, flattening at least two sides will make it fit together more securely and give better insulation value. All of this work can be done with hand tools or a chainsaw. A chainsaw is of course much faster, but some people still prefer to do it by hand, even today.

Though technically, you could build a log home directly on the ground, it is strongly recommended that you don't. Moisture in the ground will eventually cause the timbers to rot which can lead to health risks (mold and mildew) as well as structural failure. Instead, it is recommended that you construct a simple foundation on which to build your log home. This can be made simply by stacking stones together and using a simple mortar, or even clay, to bond them and fill in the gaps. Or, it can be made with either cement, or a combination of stones and cement. Even if the foundation is only one foot tall, it will keep the wood frame out of the moisture and make for a healthier, warmer, and longer lasting home.

The principles of a log home are fairly simple, but there are two major difficulties you may encounter. The first is finding logs that are straight enough. In some regions this is not a problem. Pine, and particularly Lodge Pole Pine, grows beautifully straight, but unless planted by humans, it is generally only found in colder regions. In other climates, it can take a significant effort to find trees that grow straight enough. On the subject of choosing your timber, softwoods are generally preferred. Hardwood is prone to chipping and splitting, making it much more difficult to work with and most varieties of hardwood will rot faster than say, pine or cedar.

The other difficulty, is the fireplace and chimney. Or alternately, a wood stove. A metal chimney pipe can simplify this to a degree, but as it is not natural, many people refuse to use them. Deciding where you intend to build the fireplace before any construction begins, can make things much easier. As you've no doubt seen on other homes of various styles, for a fireplace your chimney will be constructed outside of the building. Build out your foundation to make the base of the chimney. This is where it is easier if you know ahead of time where you want to build it. If doing it ahead of time, build out the chimney up to the height of the rest of the foundation. You will create a sort of pit on the outside of the foundation wall. Once you have reached the floor height, fill the pit with sand and gravel, then begin constructing the building itself.

All of this can be done with the building already constructed, it is simply easier to do ahead of time.

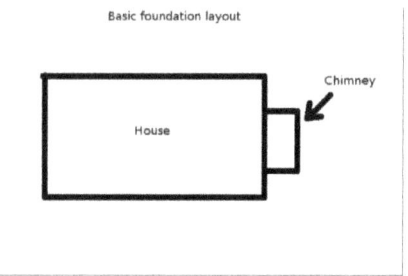

Basic foundation layout

While wood heat is undesireable to some, if you truly intend to be "off the grid" you have very few alternatives. The only feasable alternatives are electric or radiant heat. Both require vast amounts of energy no matter how efficient they are. It is unlikely your solar, wind, and other green energies will be able to keep up in the winter months.

Once the house is built, you need to cut out a hole in the wall where the fireplace is going to go. With the hole cut out, use large stones and cement to create a stone floor over your gravel filled pit and extend that floor into the house, creating the base for your hearth. Then, using wooden blocks and braces to hold everything in place, line the hole in the wall with stone and cement. Then continue building the walls of the chimney upwards. This creates the opening for the smoke to escape. You can slope in the sides to make it more narrow, but you will want an opening that is at least one foot wide. Wood bracing is strongly recommended during construction to keep the chimney straight and level. Bracing should also be used on the inside of the chimney to maintain a consistent dimension for the opening. If the chimney gets narrower towards the top, it won't ventilate as well and can cause the house to fill with smoke. Additionally, try to keep the inside of the chimney as smooth as possible. Every bulge, abnormality, or rough edge creates a place for creosote to build up, which leads to more frequent chimney sweeping and the risk of chimney fires. Once your chimney is above the roof (ideally more than one foot above) contInue building up two oposing sides while leaving the other two sides open. This allows smoke to escape out the sides when it is capped. The cap can be made with braces, stones and cement. However, if you can aquire a large enough flat stone to cover the chimney in one piece, it will be stronger and less prone to cracking or leaking. It is strongly recommended you have at least two people present for placing the cap stone as it will likely be too heavy to handle for one person on a ladder.

An alternative to this method, is to construct a cob fireplace and chimney with a log home. The design is basically the same. But, cob won't require the use of cement. Often this decision is made for you based on the material available in the area. In many places, aquiring enough stone to build a chimney would require actual quarying. Likewise, in other locations, clay or sand may be hard to come by. Ultimately, the decision is yours. Also keep in mind that wood stoves, fireplaces and all kinds of chimneys can be built in the house rather than sticking out the side. However, extending your chimney through the roof, rather than beside it, will require extensive flashings and heat resistant sealant to prevent the roof from leaking.

Whether a log home or a cob home, the roof should be given special consideration. There are many ways a roof can be constructed, but two methods in particular should be considered for an "off grid" home. Those methods are a living roof, or a roof intended for solar panels.

For a solar roof, a low pitch can prove more effective. The ideal slope of your panels will vary as the seasons change. With a low pitched roof, a simple rail system can accomodate this nicely. Build two rails across the width of the roof, attach one near the bottom of the roof and leave the other one unattached. Make the upper rail long enough to extend past the roof by a few inches on either side. Attach the bottom of the panels to the bottom rail, using hinges. Attach the top of your panels to the other rail which is still not attached to the roof. On either end of the upper rail, attach "arms" that extend downwards below the roof, about three feet in length. Lift and lower these arms until your panels are at the desired angle. Secure these arms to the roof using screws. When the seasons change and you want to adjust your panels, simply remove the screws, reposition the arms and put the screws back in. You can of course create an automated system with small motors, light sensors, etc. But, it doesn't need to be that complex to be effective.

If not using solar panels, a living roof can be quite beneficial. To prevent rot, a membrane will need to be used. After the roof is constructed, build a perimeter around the roof that is at least five inches higher than the roof. Then, place and seal the rubber membrane as per the manufacturer's instructions. Cover the membrane with at least four inches of lightly packed soil, and seed it. There are many shallow rooting, edible plants that could be grown on your roof, giving you more overall space for crops. In addition to providing more growing space, these living roofs are incredibly well insulated.

The insulation value of the soil will keep the house warmer in the winter and cooler in the summer.

The type of roof you build should most certainly be determined before construction begins. A living roof for example, is quite heavy on it's own. Depending on the square footage, just the soil can be thousands of pounds. Add a snow load to that, and your roof is supporting a massive amount of weight. Your beams and rafters will need to be bigger and stronger than they would to support a simple shingled roof with a snow load. The last thing you want to do, is to try reinforcing your roof after the fact. As far as specific load ratings, strengths, etc, there are far too many things to take into account to list it all here. That information can be found in your local building codes. However, it is complicated even further when using logs as opposed to milled lumber. If you are unsure of the dimensions and strengths your post, beams and rafters need, consult a local engineer or carpenter. NOT an architect.

Something else to consider when designing your homestead, is a root cellar. Root cellars are crucial to going off the grid. Done properly, they can prevent produce from spoiling better than a standard refrigerator, and require absolutely no energy. Root cellars are generally located under the house, but they don't have to be. A root cellar is simply a dry, dark hole in the ground. They are best made from brick or cement. Because root cellars are dug into the ground, they naturally stay cool with less temperature fluctuations than a refrigerator. Keeping your root cellar dry and dark is equally important. If you notice water on the floor or walls, locate where the water is coming in and stop it as quickly as possible. Moisture will lead to rotten food. Also, stand inside your root cellar with the door closed and make sure that no light is coming in. Even in cool, dry conditions, light can make many vegetables, potatoes for example, try to root which often makes them unedible.

If you intend to have plumbing in your house, abundant hot water can be had with no aditional energy used. To do this, you need to have a wood stove or a fireplace inside the house, not sticking out the side. If that's the case, a discarded hot water tank can be stripped of unneccessary parts such as insulation and electrical parts, and positioned against the side of your stove. One part you must be sure NOT to remove, is the pressure valve. This valve will prevent explosion if the water in the tank gets too hot. Placing the stripped down tank against the wood stove, can provide you with all the hot water you need with no electricity used. The important thing to remember with this, is not to let the tank actually touch the stove. Leave a small gap in between them, not much, just half an inch is adequate. This will keep the water hot but won't bring it to a boil. If the water starts boiling Inside the tank, and the pressure valve fails, the tank can rupture. A rupture will usually happen with explosive force and can be extremely dangerous. If, on the other hand, the water is not getting hot enough, painting the tank black will raise the temperature inside.

Another method for hot water is to use a copper coil, on or in the stove. This does work, but can be dangerous. It is very hard to control the temperature using this method and one extra piece of wood in the fire, is all it takes to make the copper coil crack from the heat and pressure.

However, if you have the skills, a low flow, low power water pump can be wired to a thermostat on the tank. This would push water through the copper pipe when the water temperature is low, and stop the flow when it's hot. This method would give you the most consistent temperatures, but does require additional energy to power the pump, as well as some type of additional pressure valve to let boiling water out of the coil.

One issue that is often overlooked when people decide to try homesteading, is waste. In general, any location where a large enough property can be aquired, will not have garbage pickup. This means you will need to transport your garbage to the local dump, yourself. But, due to climbing minimum fees at the dumps, you won't want to do this every time you fill a garbage bag. You will want to store your garbage until you have a good sized truck load. Herein lies the problem. Storing garbage attracts animals. This can endanger not only crops, but yourself as well. It is not cheap, but the best way to deal with this problem, is to invest in a bearproof dumpster. There are many distributors to be found with a quick search online. The dumpsters come in a wide variety of designs and sizes. Some even have a rubber seal around the lid to reduce smell. This is ideal as it will attract far fewer animals. Whether you purchase a dumpster or build one yourself, you will want to locate it as far away from your crops as possible. This also applies for compost.

Composting is essential for your gardening efforts if you wish to avoid chemical fertilizers. Positioning your compost far away from the garden will mean more labor when you want to apply the compost to your soil. But, compost attracts many rodents and bugs. Keeping it close to your crop may be handy, but will likely result in your entire crop being eaten by pests. The extra work of hauling compost from the far side of the property, is well worth it. On smaller properties this may not be enough, but it is certainly worth trying. One way to reduce the smell, and the number of pests, is to spread a shovel full (or two) of clean soil on top of the compost, every time you add to it. A thin blanket of soil won't be enough to prevent nearby animals from smelling the compost, but it will prevent the smell from attracting animals that are miles away. Every little bit helps. You can also plant mint around your compost (and crops too) and let it grow wild. The smell of fresh growing mint is a strong repellant for many pests, including a number of rodents.

Chapter 3: Best Animals For Homesteading

If you are interested in reducing your dependence on the outside world, then you should raise animals because the animals can provide you:

• Healthy meat and poultry without any hormones
• Fresh milk and eggs to make your morning happy
• You can get fresh cheese and butter as by-products
• The animals will bring joy to your whole family
• You can get mowed down grass and fertilizers for the plants
• It is easy to multiply them because their population can be increased easily

Animals that You can Raise
Following are some animals that you can easily raise in your farmhouse:

Raise Goats

Goats are the excellent choice to rise while living off the grid because these require low maintenance and they can take care of themselves. There will be no need to make some extra expenses because goats love to eat bushes, trees, scrub and aromatic herbs. The sheep and cattle may starve to death in the absence of a particular food, but the goats can survive easily. The goat milk is good for the elder people, patients and children having allergies to cow milk. The ulcer patients can also use goat milk. The fat and casein of the goat milk are really easy to digest as compared to the cow milk.

The goats offer lots of benefits, and they will not require anything in return. They can eat your wild plants and offer you milk. You can play with them and use their meat as well. It is quite rewarding to raise urban goats because of convenience in raising them.

There are basically six types of goats, including Nubians, Alpines, Togenburgs,

Oberhaslis, LaManchas, and Saanens. If you are looking for the best breed, then you can choose Nubian because these can give quality goat milk. These types of goats can give milk in maximum quantity.

Raising Cows

If you want to raise a cow, think twice about it because it will be your biggest responsibility in the farm. You need to arrange fodder for it and milk it twice a day. The cow dung can be used as compost can be your biggest responsibility. You need to spend more time with the cow because the cow will require your most attention. The cow will be the source of more profit because you can make cheese and butter with the milk of cows. You can sell these items in the market to earn more profit.

Raise Sheep in Your Farmhouse

The sheep are very good to keep because they can support themselves easily. They can live in the grass and become very fat. They will not make any demands from you unless the ground is covered with the snow. These are very cheap to keep and it will be good to have a native breed to the country. You can get meat and fur from sheep to make some profit.

Raise Chickens

You can raise the chicken on the healthy way by providing them enough space to flap their wings and scrap. It will be good to keep dust baths and keep them in a cage. If you want to enjoy eggs for the whole year, feed your chicken with a handful of grains in the evening and give high protein food items in the morning. They will like to eat grass and hatch little chicks. If you want to keep your garden secure, then don't leave chickens in your garden otherwise they will spoil everything.

It will be good to have a cock among your hens and give plenty of space to them in the fields and woods. The hens will constantly produce eggs, but you can also get their meat if needed. The extra supply of eggs can be sold in the market to earn some money.

Raise Geese

It is very easy to raise geese in your farmhouse because it requires low maintenance and easy to keep. The three geese in a pen with one opposite gender will live happily on the grass. You can feed those grains and keep them in your home to avoid foxes. The grain is not necessary fro geese, but you should throw the grains in the night to lure them; otherwise they will be attacked by rats and foxes. The rats can steal the eggs and young geese, but the mother goose may protect their young geese under features. The geese may start laying in the February or March.

You can keep any animal or bird in your livestock as per your convenience. You need to think about the available space and maintenance cost before selecting any bird or animal for your livestock.

Chapter 4: How Much Land

Deciding how many acres of land you are looking for -- and how much you can afford -- is one of the first things to consider. For either goal -- homesteading or small-scale farming -- you could go as small as an acre or two, or as big as many hundreds of acres. Here, you'll need to go back to your goals to figure out what amount of land will allow you to achieve those goals. For example, if you're homesteading, plan to use wood heat and be totally energy self-sufficient, you may need to add wooded acreage to your list of must-haves, so that you can provide for your own energy needs by managing a woodlot. Obviously, if you're planning to homestead in the Southwest and put up solar panels, that's a different story altogether -- you don't need that extra acreage to provide for your energy needs.
Similarly, if your goal is to start a small grass-fed beef operation, you'll need to

consider what size herd you are possibly going to have eventually, and look for a parcel of land that can support those animals.

Remoteness

How close do you want to be to town? Do you care if you're an hour's drive from a town with any kind of cultural amenities? Might you want to homestead or farm in an area that is closer to a city center for your kids' sake? These are more factors to consider.

The Internet gives you a lot more flexibility these days in terms of ordering food and supplies to remote outposts. But culturally, you're giving up quite a lot by living in a very remote area, especially if you consider your kids' need for a social life, your own desire for community and friends, and even safety and health. Even things like whether you will have neighbors within walking distance should be considered when you look at where to purchase land.

Oh, and let's not forget road maintenance. Not all land is on town- or county-maintained roads. Here the remote, privately maintained roads are called "class IV" roads. If you're looking at land on such a road, be sure to price the following services as well: gravel, grading, and other maintenance costs like plowing if you're in a snowy area.

Some places are remote enough that they don't have access to a phone line or broadband Internet, and you may have to pay to have power run to them if you aren't going to be off the grid right away. These are all things to consider as you look at the land's location.

Land Characteristics

Separate from how much acreage, the type of land is also something to consider in light of your goals. Pasture for cows is different from land used to grow vegetables. An orchard requires a certain type of land. Poultry can do well almost anywhere. These are all factors to list out on your piece of paper.

You will also want to consider factors such as natural windbreaks, drainage, local wildlife, flooding potential, and more. You may want to hire an environmental engineer to help you assess a piece of land for these types of factors.

Consider also whether there are restrictions or covenants on what you can use the land for. Can you raise any farm animal you want? Is an outhouse acceptable or must you put in a septic system for your home?

South-facing cleared land that receives at least 5 hours of direct sunlight every day is needed for growing vegetables for food. You will want level or gently sloping land unless you want to put in terraced gardens. You'll want more acreage than you think for growing all your own food as a homesteader, as you may need to rotate in cover crops to build soil fertility. If you're a small farmer who will grow vegetables for money, your land needs can vary widely depending on the type and quantity of plants you plan to grow.

An orchard, if you want to start one, requires some acreage, but can start as small as a one-half acre. For a family, a dozen or more fruit trees seems to be a rough guideline for homesteading, but this varies depending on your climate and your fruit consumption.

The quality of the soil you're buying is another thing to consider. Often, farms are abandoned because the soil was of poor quality. But, quality can be improved -- it just takes time. Having the soil tested is a smart idea when you have found a piece of property that meets all your other requirements.

Alternative Energy Needs

Wind, water (micro-hydroelectric) and solar are all possible alternative energy systems you may want to use on your small farm or homestead. What kind of land will support the type of alternative energy most suited to your climate? Will you be able to use any of these methods to generate energy with the land you're considering?

Water

If you're looking at raw land, you will probably want to have a well drilled for water. Existing farms may be using a shallow dug well from decades ago, and those can sometimes dry up. Consider the cost of well drilling - sometimes it can be significantly more expensive than you think, depending on the type of land.

And if you're going to raise livestock, you may want to look at ponds, brooks, streams -- anything that can be used to provide water for your animals.

You will, of course, also want to consider how high the water table is and if the land is prone to flooding. A seasonally flooded area can't be used for livestock for a significant portion of the year.

Access

As mentioned above, you'll need to consider how you will access your property. Is it on a maintained road? And even if the property is on a maintained road, how long of a driveway or road will you need to the spot where you want to or can build a house? Who will plow the driveway in winter?

Also look at whether there is a right of way or any other access rights going through the property.

Consider how easily a propane or oil truck can access the house, as well, if needed to provide these things for heating and cooking.

Setting Homestead Farm Goals

Whether you own your land or are still dreaming of the time when you can move to your small farm or homestead, you can set goals for what you hope to accomplish.

For many people, their vision and ideas are clear-cut. They may know already that they want to grow a small market garden, or that they want to have sheep, but not goats. Some may be clear that they want a smattering of many species of animals, a "barnyard in their backyard," just for enjoyment.

If you aren't sure yet what your overarching goals are for your small farm, ask yourself these questions.

For Money or for Pleasure

This is truly the most important question to ask. A small farm that is a business is very different from one that is a hobby farm or even for self-sufficiency. All of your decisions and planning will stem from a business perspective, even if your only goal is to sell some lettuce and eggs at the farmer's market.

Self-Sufficiency

There's a distinction between a hobby farm and a homestead. A hobby farm isn't concerned with producing a quantity of food (vegetables, fruit, dairy and/or meat) for the family. The animals and garden may produce food, but it's more a byproduct of the goal, which is to have animals and a garden for enjoyment. A homestead, or a farm whose goal is ultimately to produce most to all of its own food, look at this as the primary goal. Enjoyment of the animals and garden is still important, but the focus is shifted to self-sufficiency, and this drives decision-making.

Quality of Life

This may help you decide on your overarching goal for your small farm or homestead. For example, do you value "downtime"? You might think about starting small and slowly adding animals and garden space, so that you can adjust the balance of work and play more easily. Do you enjoy farm work as downtime? You might jump in more quickly, knowing that you're less likely to get overwhelmed.

How much are you willing to put off or forego other activities and things to expand your small farm? If you could afford to get a dairy cow but that meant giving up your weekly night out, would it be worth it to you? These are things to think about and analyze as you consider the quality of life questions.

Overarching Life Philosophy

Yep, that one's a doozy. But it's something to consider deeply as you move forward with your small farm venture. If you haven't grown up in a farming tradition, and your attitude is that you are "dabbling" in farming, you are much more likely to give up when things get tough as they inevitably will.

Spend some time now to think about the "big picture" things that are driving the decision to farm. Maybe the belief that we need to live more lightly on the earth, and that peak oil and the food crisis are bearing down on us, is driving your decision to homestead. Perhaps it's just reconnecting with a sense of contentment and well-being that you felt like a kid on your grandparents' farm that you're looking to recapture with a hobby farm in your retirement.

Whatever the philosophy that is underpinning your decision to farm, write it down. It may be more than one thing - that's fine. Having your philosophy written down can help when you get lost in the details. You have something to turn to, a tangible reminder of why you're doing this.

Tips for the Beginning Homesteader

Are you new to homesteading or thinking about establishing your own homestead? Learn from others and avoid repeating their mistakes. Take a look at some of expert homesteader best tips for those considering to start a self-sufficient homestead.

Set Realistic Goals

Many people who get frustrated and overwhelmed with homesteading take on more than they can reasonably handle, then feel overwhelmed and stretched too thin. Set your sights on a couple of really solid goals each season instead of scattering your efforts across many goals. You may end up fragmented and frazzled.

Is It Right for You?

Are you really cut out to be a homesteader? Think long and hard before embarking on what is ultimately a labor of love. Be prepared to put in long, tough hours of physical labor, often painful and uncomfortable, for the sheer joy of being able to provide for your own needs. If you have grown up in modern society, as most of us have, this can be a huge adjustment and not one that most people can make easily.

Plan for Some Income

Although you might initially fantasize that you can provide everything you need for yourself and your family and never spend a penny, that is not realistic. You will need to consider that there will be expenses you will have that will require money, especially as you transition to a self-sustaining homestead.

Also, evaluate how you like to live. Do you enjoy going to restaurants or going out dancing? Do you like to travel or attend cultural events? You will need some income to afford the things in life that cannot be bartered or made yourself.

Eschew Debt

Borrowing money goes against every principle that underlies the goal of self-sufficiency. People who want to homestead generally want to be able to disengage from the money economy and work as little as possible in exchange for money. Instead of using money, homesteaders grow their own food and perhaps barter for things like clothing and other necessary items.

Keep Your Expenses Low

This becomes important when considering your homestead property (most people who homestead want to buy their own land or house). Will you buy land with cash and build a house on it yourself with cash as well? Or will you buy a house already built on some acreage? If you are considering taking on a mortgage to buy your homestead property, how will you pay your mortgage? Do you plan to pay it off over a shorter time frame than 30 years?

Also, consider how your homestead will be heated and cooled and how electricity will be provided. Using sustainable energy sources like solar, wind, or geothermal can reduce your expenses significantly. Many homesteaders refuse to be "on the grid," wanting to provide their own electricity as a critical part of their self-sufficiency goals. You will need to devote some time to decide how you will provide for these needs on your own homestead.

Embrace Simplicity and Give Up on Aesthetics

This is important. As a homesteader, you have one goal: self-sufficiency. The hours that you spend making things pretty are hours that you could be doing functional things to further your goal of self-sufficiency.

If you put pressure on yourself to make your homestead look like it belongs in "Better Homesteads and Gardens," while doing all the things needed in a day to maintain a homestead, it is an unrealistic goal. You are likely to get frustrated and overwhelmed when you do not succeed.

Let go of any remaining attachment to things looking neat and together. It will help you achieve more.

At the same time, if you are chugging along, happily advancing toward your ultimate goal of self-sufficiency, and not stressed, and able to keep things organized and tidy to boot, then great. The point is to not stress out over it.

A life of luxury and glamour is not in the cards for a homesteader. Homesteading is all about the idea that trading time for money does not serve you as well as using your time to provide for your needs directly. Simple living, or living lightly on the earth, means reducing one's possessions and expenditures and learning to be satisfied with just meeting your needs, and letting go of wants and consumption.

Time Worked Equals Self-Sufficiency

If you resent the time spent tending animals, canning food, and chopping wood—then homesteading is not for you. Instead, consider a hobby farm where your goal is just to enjoy the parts of farming that you do not resent, without self-sufficiency as the ultimate goal. Or maybe a small farm business is the right choice, where your focus is on earning money as well as farming.

Divorce time from money in your mind. Sure, you could have worked for maybe $15 an hour, but instead, you just worked the equivalent of $5 an hour by raising your own chickens. The whole point is that you worked for yourself, on your own terms, and you are building something that runs deeper than trading your time for an hourly wage.

Roll With the Punches

Humor is a good thing. Laugh daily. Do not get on a high horse about homesteading and think you are superior to everyone else. When things go wrong when the chickens start pooping all over the front steps and foxes start attacking your hens, try to keep perspective.

You will need to take it easy on yourself and be OK when you do not reach your goals as quickly as you thought. If needed, sit down and retool your plan to reflect new goals and new timelines. Everything can be adjusted. Enjoy the process of gaining self-sufficiency a little bit at a time.

Chapter 5: Homestead Life Hack

#4 - Milling Lumber

"We are all fed from hundreds and thousands of hands. Often we do not know whose they are nor how they work. Only a few of us ever visualize the hands that grope in the coal mines or push levers in the mills or handle axes in the lumber camp."

- Louis MacNeice

"Houston, we have a problem," my mobile phone ringtone declared from my night stand.

I grasped the phone, "Jim," I said. "What's up?" I knew it was my manager calling, because it was the ringtone I assigned to him. I glanced at the clock. It was 2 am.

"It's all hands on deck..." he said. I could hear that he was calling from his truck. "I'm heading to the site, Brian is on his way in as well and Dave is monitoring the systems from home. We're in island mode. All gens are running. When can you get here?"

At the time, I was the construction manager for the data center technical team. When things went wrong with operations, I always jumped in and helped. "I'm leaving now..." I said. "I'll be on site in about 30 minutes."

With that, I jumped from my bed, slipped on my jeans, a shirt, socks and my boots. I grabbed my phone, truck keys and headed for the door.

My garage door opened to the sound of the pounding rain. It was bad. Winds were gusting between 50 and 70 miles per hour. I bolted for my truck.

I threw it in reverse and sped backwards. I put it in drive and started up my driveway. My heart stopped.

Three trees, about 27" thick at chest height leaned across my driveway. I backed up.

There is a small side road out of my property as well. I threw my truck into 4-wheel drive and started through the mud.

I made it 25 feet when I realized another tree of the same size lay across the trail.

Growing up in North Central Pennsylvania, it was common to heat with wood. I had spent many years cutting logs into firewood as a child. My father believed firmly in forced child labor (just ask my brothers). That is where I first learned to use a chainsaw.

As I grew older, I decided that it would be nice to own one. So, I received a small bonus at work and purchased a 16" Poulan chainsaw.

Now, for the everyday home owner, that saw will work just fine. Mine cut well, but it would never idle and would always shut off. I always had to restart it if I set it down between cuts.

All of the trees that came crashing down on that stormy night, needed to be removed.

And, quite honestly, I was not the man to do it. There was so much tension in those trees that a wrong cut could cause the tree to snap and kill you. So, I called in a professional.

During my discussion with him, I asked him to cut the logs in 6 to 8 foot lengths and to set them on the side of the driveway. He was more than happy to do so.

The logs lay there for 6 months. My wife asked me several times what I planned to do with them.

Finally, I said, "I want to get a mini-lumber mill and mill my own lumber."

She looked at me out of the corner of her eye as if to say, you're kidding me, right?

"I'm serious." I said. "I've looked up everything I need. I can buy a Granberg mini-mill that will fit a chainsaw for about $250."

"That's not bad." She said, starting to buy into the idea. "Will the chainsaw you have still work?"

I shook my head. "I want to buy a professional grade saw."

"How much?"

"I found a Husqvarna 572. I need the 32" bar for those trees."

"Why?" She said, "The trees are only 27" wide."

"I know, but everything I read online said that you will lose 5 to 6 inches with the rig."

Improvise, Adapt and Overcome:

I bought the Granberg mini-mill and the Husqvarna 572, and let me say this…

It is one of the greatest things I have ever done.

The saw and the mini-mill paid themselves off within a matter of 6 months. Once you understand the mechanics of the system and how you set up the saw on the mill, you can rip right through the logs.

Since purchasing the system, I have milled live edge lumber which I sell. I have also rough cut 2x4's, 4x4's, 6X6's and even 8x8's. I sell them as fireplace mantels and use them when building projects around my homestead.

I would highly recommend to any homesteader, if you have access to timber, you definitely need to have a system to mill lumber.

You will never regret it.

Here are photos of the materials and my projects:

Chapter 6: Introduction To Indoor Gardening

Winter has come and the cold weather has posed its challenge to your garden. How do you keep up with your self-sustainability practices when you don't have an outdoor garden for the season? The answer is pretty simple, and it can be applied to any home, for any season, too! Instead of confining your garden to your back or front yard, why not extend your productive soil inside your house?

What is Indoor Gardening?

As the name implies, indoor gardening is the practice of growing plants inside the confines of your house. This might sound messy and complicated, but with a little bit of creativity and common sense, you'll find that Indoor Gardening is both a great alternative and companion for regular organic gardening.

What are the limits of Indoor Gardening?

Again, space is an issue here, but this can be easily remedied by using a few innovative ideas. Since your house has furniture, and people are constantly moving in and out of rooms, your pots and plants must be relatively small, compared to those that you would usually grow outside in your backyard.

What do you need for Indoor Gardening?

You need to carefully pick out your seeds or seedlings for your Indoor Garden. If you have some seeds leftover from your backyard garden, you can use those to jumpstart your indoor garden venture. You can also take a short trip to gardening centers and grocery stores for different seeds taken from organic plants. Aside from your seeds, seedlings or pots, you will also need a small watering can (though a pitcher or spray bottle will do just fine), gloves, a small trowel (or a spoon, if you are working with really small plants and pots), and of course, a good helping of compost.

Tips for Starting an Indoor Garden

1. Look around your house for a suitable place to put your plants. They will need sunlight, fresh air, and they should be far away from pets or small children. Once you find such a place, dedicate a few hours to cleaning it up and preparing it for your garden.

2. Decide on what plants you want to grow. Are you going to stick with culinary herbs? Or are you going to add a few earthy vegetables that can be grown in small pots, maybe even add flowers and ornamentals, too?

3. Prepare all the materials you will need for planting. Remember to read seed packet labels very well, and research how to grow them properly. Also, be attentive to the amount of water you give your plants. You should also keep in mind that they will not grow as big as the crops in your outdoor garden so lower your expectations a bit.

Ideas for an Effective Indoor Garden

1. Use old plastic egg cartons for starting herb seed containers. Once the herbs begin to sprout, you can use yogurt cups,

or ice cream tubs to hold them until maturity.

2. Look for an old shoe rack, or build one out of recycled metal or wood. You can use the shelves to maximize the space of your indoor garden. Plant racks also double as a tool cabinet!

3. You can also hang small plants from the ceiling, especially those ornamentals that thrive in higher places.

Chapter 7: Homestead Life Hacks

#5, 6, 7 & 8 - Improvise, Adapt and Overcome
"No battle plan ever survives contact with the enemy."

-Helmuth von Moltke the Elder

I sat back in the black chair.Her office was very comfortable.It was familiar.It was safe.

"You know," I said."I am amazed at the ability of soldiers to improvise, adapt and overcome."

She nodded.

"Let me give you a specific example..."I paused."When we were in Iraq, we didn't have cold water..."

The desert wind blew sharp and dry against our faces on that day.It was approximately 1300 hours.We stood, as we usually did, around the tanks on the tank line.There wasn't much to do and so we started goofing off while no one was watching.

I watched as a friend of mine took some non-potable water, drenched a sock that he had retrieved from his duffle bag and then stretched the wet sock over a bottle of drinking water.

He hoisted himself onto the hull of the tank and then set the bottle on top of the turret.

It was hot that day.I don't remember how hot it was, maybe 100 or 110 degrees F.

It was a dry heat.

We all just kind of looked at him and dismissed him as another CDAT (That's what we were so affectionately called by our infantry counterparts.CDATs... Computerized Dumb Ass Tankers).

We continued to goof off.

An hour later, I watched as my friend returned to the bottle of water, slipped the sock off, took a sip, smacked his lips and let out a big "Aaaahhhhhh..."

He looked at us and smiled.

I looked at him."What's that?" I said nodding my head in an upward motion.

"Water," he responded with a smart ass smirk.

He handed it to me.

I grabbed the bottle and I was shocked.

It was cold.

How the heck did that happen? I thought.

And then suddenly, I realized ...I didn't care how it happened, nor did I care about the magic behind it.It was 110 degrees outside and I was tired of drinking lukewarm water.

"Show me what you did."I demanded.

He smiled. "Get a sock from your duffle bag and bring it back to me."

I ran to my tank and returned with a sock.

I watched him pour water over the sock, slip the sock over the bottle and place it on top of the tank.

"Now, all you have to do is wait." He said and walked back to the other guys.

I stood by the tank.Waiting... Just waiting...

And I waited... impatiently... for 30 minutes... until I couldn't wait any longer.

I seized the bottle and quickly drank.

As soon as the bottle left my lips, I sputtered to myself, "You've got to be kidding me. The water's colder."

I felt like a caveman who had just discovered fire. I was so excited, that I was almost dancing a tribal dance, around my bottled water with a wet sock over the top, praising the gods above for deliverance from the heat.

I just stood there in amazement with the Grinch's grin on my face.

My VA Psychologist smiled at me, as she leaned forward.

"But that's not all," I continued. "Conner (my son) wanted to do a science fair project. I suggested to him that we could do 'The Cooling of Water through Evaporation'. And we did that."

She nodded.

"You won't believe this…He won first place."

She looked at me, "That is so cool. I love the fact that you revisited that."

I reached for my phone to show her a picture of my son with his first place trophy. After sharing the photo with her, I sat back down.

"Now, I want to read you something that I wrote." My thumb swiped the screen of my phone looking for my Notes application.

I keep all of my notes on my phone. I travel a lot for work. It's nice to be on a plane and to be able to pick up my iPhone, open the "Notes" application and capture my thoughts. It's convenient.

I opened the app and read the following to her:

"Conner won first place and I am ecstatic about that. It is a true testament to the ability of the

American Soldier to improvise, adapt and overcome...

To achieve nothing more than a simple pleasure in life... To drink cold water on a hot day."

Improvise, Adapt and Overcome:

I learned a lot in Iraq. I learned about loyalty, honor and brotherhood.

But there was one skill that we all relied on...Our ability to improvise, adapt and overcome.

That is a skill that I continue to use everyday of my life.

So... following are some of the ways I have improvised, adapted and overcame.I hope you find them as useful as I did and still do.

Tomatoes Grown Upside Down

This is one of my favorites...I was watching a YouTube video one night and came across a young fellow that was sharing how he grew vegetables in his container garden in Mumbai.The best part was this, he was reusing plastic containers so they wouldn't have to be thrown out.Here are the steps to making your own:

1. Get a tomato plant.

2. Get an old orange juice or milk container.

3. Prune the tomato plant so there are only leaves in the top portion.You can't have any branches on the sides because they won't fit through the top of the container.

4. Cut off the bottom of the container about 1" up from the bottom.

5. Drill four small holes in the sides of the container opposite each other about ¼" from the bottom.

6. Put wire from one hole to the other that is opposite and fasten it. Do the same with the other hole. This will act as your hanger.

7. Feed the tomato plant into the container and place the vine through the top of the container.

8. Turn the container upside down and fill with soil.

9. Water heavily.

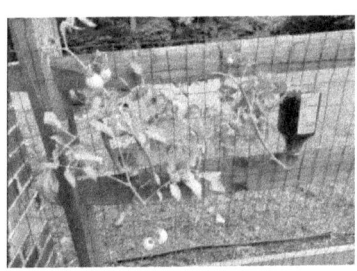

Two Containers From One

As we ventured into container gardening, we realized that it can get very expensive, very quickly. We walked through our basement and I saw some old cracked

plastic bins.I thought, what if I cut them in half and added a bottom to one of the halves and drilled holes in the bottom of the other half?
And that's what I did.
As you can see, my peas turned out very well.

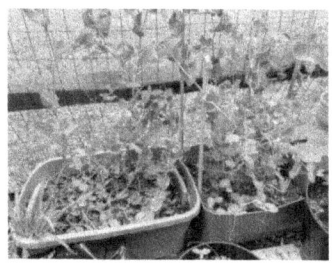

Trash To Treasure
A buddy of mine was moving to his new home.I have known this man for a long time.He is a dear friend so I offered to help.
As we neared the end of the day, he had dis-assembled his daughter's toddler bed and was taking the wood to the trash.
"Whoa, whoa, whoa..." I said. "What are you doing?"

He looked at me puzzled."Um, throwing it out."
I looked at him."I'll take it." I said.With that, I threw it into the bed of my F150 and headed for home.
I cut up that bed and made containers.To make the wood go further, I spread out the cross boards.I then used old garbage bags as the liners, cut slits into the bottoms so water could leach out and I planted them.They worked great.

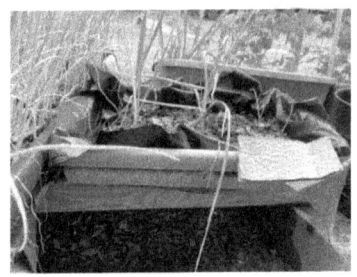

The Art and Science of Composting
Yeah...not much science here for me.
Notice I said, "for me".
There is some serious science behind composting.I read articles, watched YouTube videos and absorbed any other

composting information that I could get my hands on.All of the science behind composting was almost intimidating and was delaying me starting to compost out of fear of failure (See the Prologue).

I decided that I just needed to move forward.After all of my research, I came up with a simple formula that works for me.But first, let's define a couple of things.

"Green Material" - This is anything that would come out of your kitchen or it may be your grass clippings.It is typically plant material that was recently harvested.

"Brown Material" - This would be anything that has been dead for some time and is brown.Some examples would be leaves, wood, etc.

My formula for composting is simple:

I use a 2:1 ratio of Brown Materials to Green Materials by volume.

What does that mean?

Well, simply this... For every bucket of Green Material, I mix it with 2 buckets of Brown Material.

Now I needed compost bins.

I did more research.I decided on the 3 Bin Compost System.So, I built three compost bins out of small sticks because it was free[5].The 3 Bin System is simple.The first bin is for fresh compost (Green and Brown Materials mixed in the ratio I use).One month later, I move it to the second bin.I then put the fresh compost in the first bin.In the second month, I transfer the 2nd bin to the 3rd bin, the 1st bin to the 2nd bin and I fill the first bin with the fresh compost.

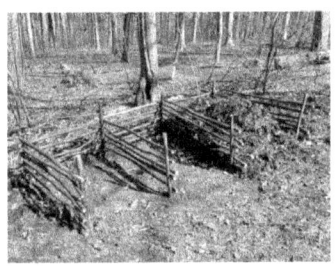

In the fourth month (if the compost is ready) I will "Top Dress" my raised beds.This means that I place a thin layer of the compost on top of my planting beds.This opens up the 3rd bin and allows me to repeat the process.

I built my bins out of sticks on my property.

Chapter 8: The Importance Of Seed Saving

Nowadays, people often take seeds for granted. After all, with the grocery stores and gardening centers, it is easy to assume that there is a near infinite supply of seeds readily available. However, in the early ages of agriculture, families would select and save the best seeds from their crops for the next generation, hence the term heirloom crops. This tradition of seed saving is still alive, and is very much relevant to worldwide food security.

What is seed saving?

Seed saving is the art and practice of selecting seeds from crops that possess certain characteristics like sturdiness, abundant crop yield, and high pest resistance. Instead of discarding the seeds you pick up from your garden, seed saving encourages that you label them properly, and stow them away until the next planting season.

Why is seed saving important?

Caring for and saving the seeds of the next crop generation is a symbol of the people's unity with the earth. It is an act of respect and reverence for the soil that yields crops that then feed people all over the globe. Seed saving helps increase food security both in small families and on an international scale. This is especially true for heirloom seeds that have been kept in certain families for several generations.

Seed saving provides an opportunity for people to reconnect with the earth, and recognizes that genetically modified seeds are still weaker strains compared to what Mother Nature designs. If all urban mini farmers made a pledge to collect and save seeds from their garden and surrounding areas, then the world would have a better chance of increasing crop diversity and strength.

Where should you go for rare or heirloom seeds?

If you want to help in the propagation of rare or heirloom seeds, it would be best if sought families who have been sowing and planting a specific crop type for generations. They are likely to have saved several good seeds, and would be more than happy to trade some of those seeds with you, on the condition that you also actively engage in the act of seed saving.

How do you go about seed saving?

In your garden, you can be very meticulous about which plants are crossed with each other. Always choose the strong plants' seeds for next year's season. Pay close attention to the positive and negative characteristics of all your crops, and try to isolate the weak strains from the strong strains.

Outside of your garden, you can keep a close eye on the ground for fallen seeds that you can plant, grow and share with others. You can also donate to seed saving institutions, or help spread awareness to your fellow urban mini farmers.

Chapter 9: Maintaining Your Vegetable Garden

Vegetables require pretty much the same amount of care as ornamental plants, sometimes even less. But they certainly aren't as forgiving of neglect. Vegetable plants use a significant amount of energy to bloom and produce fruits that do not get to mature before they get harvested. A vegetable plant sets fruit so that it can produce more seeds. Still, we often end up harvesting the vegetables before the seeds become fully-formed. This can be very stressful for your vegetable plants; so, it is vital that you provide them exactly what they need and more to keep them in good health and vigor for maximum production. Neglect of your vegetable plants will often result in lower yields and poor-quality crops as a result of pest problems. The guidelines we will be discussing below will help keep your vegetables healthy as they grow along the season to give you a high-yield return on investment.

The first guideline is to water your vegetables regularly. Watering is an essential part of gardening, and the importance cannot be overstated or understated. Regular water is just as important to your plants as sunlight exposure. This means that you must give your plants at least one or more inches of water each week, and more when the weather is exceptionally hot. Without regular water, your vegetables won't fill out as they should, and some, such as tomatoes, will crack and burst open if suddenly showered with water after being denied for a while. Since you can't always expect rainfall to help you, it is better to install a drip irrigation system if you have the means. Most of the new systems on the market are easy to install, and they are very affordable. You will be able to save money on your water bill as well, because the water from your irrigation system goes directly to the vegetables' roots, making it almost impossible for you to lose water to evaporation. If you don't want to install a drip irrigation system, you can locate your garden near a reliable water source, such as a water spigot. Watering is much easier when you don't have to drag the hose out. Just as you have learned, you have to regularly get rid of excess seedlings to ensure that your garden remains very healthy. This is especially important when the plants are being sown directly from the seeds. This process is called thinning and is an essential part of vegetable garden maintenance. Many gardeners find it difficult to sacrifice their seedlings, but leaving all the sprouted and unwanted seedlings to grow closer to your healthy plants can stunt their growth and reduce the garden yield at the end of the season. Once true leaves come out of the plants, remove the seedlings to ensure that the vegetables remain at the required spacing distance. If you can't get rid of the extra seedlings without affecting the roots of the remaining plants, simply get rid of the seedlings at the soil line. Let the strongest seedlings remain.

Staking the plants is also a maintenance task that you must regularly perform at the start of the gardening season. Tall and climbing plants such as cucumbers require you to stake or trellis them. The best thing is to do the staking during the planting time. If you don't do it until the plants have grown beyond staking, you might end up injuring the plant roots. So, the staking of the vegetable plants should be done early in the season. Later on, you will need to prune suckers if you have some tomatoes in your garden. Pruning tomato suckers involves getting rid of the growth that takes place in the place between the stem and branch. If you leave the suckers to grow, they may end up becoming other stems with flowers, branches, fruit, and other suckers, which will all be competing for the same nutrients with your original tomato plants.

Veggies don't like it when you leave them to compete with weeds for the little food and water they have. Each gardening season starts on a blank slate after you ready the garden beds. Therefore, you must keep up with the weeds as soon as you have planted your vegetables. Doing this will help ensure that your crops stay in the best shape. If you get rid of weeds as soon as they appear regularly, it will never get to the point where they are out of your control. In addition to removing weeds from your garden, you must also remove nearby weeds along the surrounding pathways and the grass around your garden. If you allow the surrounding weeds to go to seed, they may just end up taking over your garden. Keeping weeds in check right from the start of the gardening season is one way to ensure you won't need to use herbicides later in the hotter climate.

Mulching is one of the most important tasks that you must perform for your plants to stay healthy. Mulching your plants help suppress the growth of weeds, cools your plants' roots, and saves water. When the plants become dense enough, they can even serve as their own mulch. The best type of mulch for vegetable gardens is seed-free straws. It is good as a cover, and also easy to push aside when it is planting time. Plus, you can turn it into good soil once the harvesting season ends. An extra perk of mulching is that spiders love to feast on garden pests while hiding in the straws.

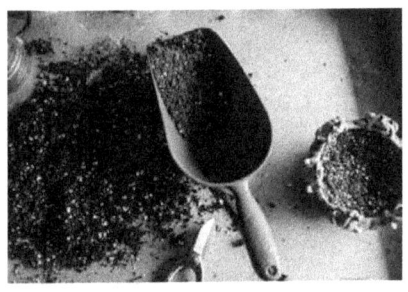

Finally, make sure you take steps to enrich the soil. Vegetables feed heavily, which is why you should mix in some organic matter into your garden every year before you plant. Furthermore, you should dress in the more organic matter once or twice while the growing season is still going strong. Of course, different plants have different needs, which means you should take note of the fertilizing guidelines that come with the seed packets or seedlings.

Organic plant foods release slowly, and they can help your plants stay fed all through the season. If you choose to go for a water-soluble fertilizer, ensure that the garden is watered well before you apply it to the soil.

Since getting great soil in your garden takes so much hard work, it is only reasonable for you to keep it the same way even at the end of the season. An easy technique for enriching the soil and keeping it protected after the season is over is to plant some green manure crops in the soil during fall and then mix it in with the soil once spring arrives. Examples of crops that are excellent for this purpose are cover crops such as alfalfa, ryegrass, and clover. All of these crops are green manure crops that can very well improve soil condition and structure and provide the beneficial microbes in the soil with nutrients, resulting in a richer and healthier soil for the next gardening season.

Chapter 10: How To Make A Living Homesteading

So you want to live self-sufficiently off the land?

Leading a homestead lifestyle requires a serious commitment on the individual's part which may include a sizable investment of the land itself.

Can the homesteading lifestyle provide an income too?

We think it can.

So the question we are attempting to answer is how to make a living homesteading?

A lot of the young people have been moving into rural areas setting up homesteads.

They take the example of their parents who grew up on large tracts of land in the rural areas.

They are preparing food in the traditional manner and basically living in a manner which utilizes minimal resources.

Here are possible income sources which will help you make a living, earn some extra money and even make the land pay for itself.

Beekeeping

Beekeeping is a fascinating hobby that many people turn into a business.

It doesn't take a lot of space, and there are many months when there is little work you will have to do which will enable you to market your business or take on other projects.

Before starting out, you may think there is only honey and honey-related products to sell.

Yet, when it comes to beekeeping, there are many income streams.

When you are starting out and learning, you will likely be drawn to some things more than others.

Perhaps you will be interested in how to breed queens or to maintain hives.

You can sell starter colonies and beehive products (including wax and starter jelly).

There's even photography, activism, science, bee removal, bee products and equipment, education, and more.

Or maybe you just want to keep bees for fun.

Make Money Selling Timber

If you have purchased a piece of land that is heavily wooded, then that in itself is a huge opportunity to earn money.

Timber companies will pay you good money to come and clear your land for you.

All you need to do is inform them that you have standing timber which you are ready to sell.

This sale can be either to large companies or even individuals.

There are always people looking to purchase firewood and you can cater to these people.

Make Money Selling Rocks

If your land has a lot of rocks then that can too be a source of income as there are people who are interested in buying all kinds of rocks.

A simple website to advertise the rocks found on your property can see a surprising amount of interest in what most people see no value in.

Make Money Selling Livestock

Livestock is reared on homesteads for the purpose of food and can be a source of income too.

There are auctions in most small towns for livestock of good breed.

These animals can be raised at your homestead and then later sold for profit.

Miniature cattle breeds are often the perfect choice for a compact farming space.

They can provide milk and later, meat.

Make Money Selling Eggs

Chicken and duck eggs are always in demand wherever your homestead may be.

These can serve as a steady source of income.

Quail eggs too go for a tidy sum and it may not be a bad idea to raise quails along with chicken and ducks.

Make Money Selling Produce

If the land is amenable to it then you can do small scale farming on it too.

It requires time, patience and skill but it pays off well in the long run.

The produce from the land can be sold at local farmers markets.

More and more people are shopping at these markets as the trend to eat local grows.

If you are short on space, consider a DIY hydroponics system.

Other sources of income

Apart from all of these you can always sell your skills that you have gathered as you set up your own homestead.

Even inventory that you may have purchased can leased out or rented out to make extra money.

Homesteading school

As the concept of homesteading is spreading across the United States, more and more people are interested in acquiring the necessary skills that will let them live off the land in a wholesome and self reliant manner.

It is to impart the skills required to run your own homestead that a number of homesteading schools are cropping up across the country.

We take a closer look at the skills that you can learn at these schools as well as list out some of the better ones across the country.

A good way to adjust to some of the change that you will face as well as learn some of the skills that you will need when you take the decision to run your own homestead is to join a homesteading school.

Most of these homesteading schools have been started by pioneers of the return to this movement.

They want to make the path that they followed easier for other to follow.

There are a number of established homesteads that have hands-on courses that allow to you to get a feel of the life firsthand as well as learn the necessary skills.

It is important to develop these skills as you work as they also can be a source of income to you in the future.

Workshops and learning on farms

Kimberly Coburn who has started Homestead Atlanta shared that she realized a number of people want to experience the fulfillment that she has by starting their own homestead.

Her school is not rigid about curriculum that they follow.

Most of the learning is practical and hands-on.

The purpose is to teach as many skills as possible in the allotted time so that a wholesome and economically viable lifestyle is possible for the 'students' that pass out from there.

The classes for these schools too can take place at a different location every time.

It can be a discussion at a restaurant or a beekeeping class at a bee farm.

The approach is low-resource by intention.

Some people prefer to take workshops at functioning farms.

These workshops are becoming more and more common across the country now and can start from as little $25 per session.
All kinds of people attend these schools and workshops, not necessarily beginners.
Learning homesteading skills
A number of people took the plunge into homesteading and then realized that there are some skills that they needed to polish or learn from scratch.
These schools have started receiving help in the form of fiscal support as well as access to facilities by corporate players in the field.
Kimberly's school had a tie up with Georgia organic that allowed her to expand the scope and reach of her program much beyond what she had possible imagined when she started out.
A simple web search for these schools reveals a map of the United States with the homesteading schools in your area marked out.

If you are considering a shift to this lifestyle then it may be a prudent idea to attend one of these schools and acquire the necessary knowledge that will allow you to make a seamless switch.

There is so much to consider when deciding whether to homestead:

Consider the move on your family and possibly being away from extended family

Year-round work it will take, in all types of weather, to make your family self-sufficient

Cost to uproot your life and move (if necessary)

Can you keep your job and start projects on the side

Consider the schooling options available if you have children.

Take the time to understand what is homesteading all about before you take this huge lifestyle change into consideration.

Investigate a homesteading school to help. And it is possible to make a living homesteading, but everyone has to be "on board."

You can start small with something that interests you, and grow from there.

Chapter 11: Backyard Homesteading

The backyard homesteading movement is about sustainability, self sufficiency, vintage skills and reclaiming a vibrant part of our history well that is what it means to me.Your reasons might be very different.Whatever your reasons I encourage you to start – the hardest step you'll take is the first one.

Backyard Homesteading addresses the needs of many people who want to take control of the food they eat and the products they use--even if they live in a urban or suburban house on a typical-size lot. It shows homeowners how to turn their yard into a productive and wholesome "homestead" that allows them to grow their own fruits and vegetables, and raise farm animals.

STEPS INTO BACKYARD HOMESTEADING

Some call it backyard homesteading but you may have heard other names like, urban homesteading, suburban homesteading or backyard farming. But the basics of backyard homesteading are the same – taking the space you have and raising food on it and reclaiming vintage skills.

It's funny that in 2014 it has become a somewhat trendy thing to do; as if it's a revolutionary idea. But, in truth, this is really taking a concept that has been part of our lives until the last few decades and making it work in today's home. From the meat rabbits of the great depression to the victory gardens of the World Wars; backyard homesteading has been a tried and true way of life.

Start a garden

This can feel challenging if you've never gardened before.Don't fear,it is really as easy as finding out what grows in your area and when, then start planning.Check with your local extension office for a planting calendar. My main gardening style is Square Foot Gardening – less space and more veggies!I started with 1 4×4 garden box and now I have 8 – add as you're feeling comfortable and confident.

If you're in an apartment consider container gardening.I use containers, like self-watering buckets and fabric pots, to extend my growing space onto my porch.I have had wonderful success using these buckets for peppers, tomatoes and even kale.But I don't use them in the summer because the summer heat in Phoenix makes the root base too hot. Remember to buy good, non-gmo, organic seeds!And good soil – a strong, healthy base is essential.

Start Composting

Composting has so many benefits less trash, healthier soil, etc.And it really isn't the daunting task you might think it is.You can even build your own trash can composter (seriously if I can, you can).Then start adding kitchen scraps, bunny droppings, coffee grounds and even egg shells.Mix in a bit of leaves, grass clippings and you're off to the races! It isn't rocket science...more like biology.

I'm sure your first thought will be chickens, and they are great. Chickens provide much more than eggs.Their waste can be composted, they'll work your compost if you let them and they are natural pest control.Unfortunately we all don't have the space for them in our backyards and not all cities allow them.

Another awesome option is quail.The Coturnix quail only needs 1 square foot of space, though more is appreciated.Hens will start laying around 8 weeks of age and generally lay an egg a day.You'll need about 3-4 of their eggs to equal one chicken egg but boy are they worth it; creamy and delicious!

Quail hens are virtual noise free – unlike chickens who sing their egg song loud & proud. Now the roos are a bit nosier, and I was so over ours after about a week.But you don't need a rooster for yummy eggs. You can keep your quail inside in cages but they do great on the ground as cage-free birds too.

Raise some Backyard Meat

The best meat you'll ever eat is the one you raise.Why?You, as the producer, decide the environment, quality of life and feed that animal receives. Now, chances are, you're not going to be raising a cow or a pig in your backyard...but there are other options.

Chickens – not a bad choice but if you can keep chickens then you'll probably want layers versus meat birds.The space and time required for meat chickens can make them problematic in an ordinary backyard.Because of this I'm not going to go into much on chickens for this article.

Quails – an excellent choice for poultry meat.Hatch to butcher is about 8 weeks and won't require much space.Quail are also much easier to process as well; a sharp pair of scissors are all you really need.Most people don't pluck their quail either just simply skin them and they are ready to go.If you're serious about raising quail for a meat source you'll want to consider getting an incubator instead of buying chicks from someone else.The incubator will quickly pay for itself and may make the rooster worth his noise (you may want to get your neighbor some eggs/meat).

Rabbits –the other white meat. Seriously though, rabbits are an excellent meat source for the backyard (apartment) homesteader. They reproduce rapidly and provide an excellent lean white meat at about 8 – 12 weeks, depending on the breed. A single doe can produce a 1,000 times her weight in meat every year; you'll never see those kind of results from any other livestock! A breeding trio could easily keep a family of 4 stocked up on rabbit meat for entire year. Processing takes about 15 minutes start to finish and the cull is quick. Keeping rabbits will be great for your garden too – rabbit droppings are easy compost additions!

Chapter 12: Vital Equipment For Homesteaders

There are five important homesteading tools and you should have them with you so that you can create a better living setup in the wilderness.

Knives with Fixed Blades

You need a durable and versatile knife with a fixed blade because you have to make traps, snares and remove the skin of animals. This knife will help you to cut smaller twigs, vegetables, and fruits. You can use a stone to maintain the better structure and sharpness of the blade. You should keep it clean and wrap in a moisture absorbent sheet to keep it in a good shape. The moisture can be the reason of rusting and corrosion so makes sure to use oil on the blade to keep it secure. Keep it always sharp because a sharp knife is better to use as compared to a dull knife. You should learn how to sharpen the blades and knives.

Axes or Hatchets

The small and versatile axes are used to butcher animals and kill snakes. These can protect you from animals and other external factors. Just like a knife, keep its blade completely dry and apply some oil before keeping it in a secure place. You can use a sandpaper to remove any rust from the surface. A light lubricant spray is available to protect the blade of your axe. Store your tool in a sheath or waterproof cloth to protect it from moisture.

Saws

It is a special tool that is required to cut woods, branches, and twigs. You can use it to get wood for the construction of wooden furniture and buildings. You can construct small storage huts and cut firewood. Keep it clean because the debris can make its cutting surface dull. A little kerosene is good to protect your saw from external elements. After cleaning it, carefully check the teeth of the saw and replace any damaged blade. The use of damaged blade is dangerous and can hurt you while working. Great the head of the saw and then keep it away from moisture to avoid rusting.

Machetes

It is just like a large knife that will help you to do the lighter job. Its blade is sharp and can do lots of cutting jobs. You can clean bushes and cut branches and logs for the fire. You should protect its blade by applying oil on it. You should store it in a dry place to avoid any rusting and deterioration. The sharp blade can do a good job as compared to a dull blade.

Backpacks

It is another important tool for Homesteading because you have to keep all important items secure. You have to buy a reliable backpack with sufficient space to protect all your tools. Make sure to buy a backpack with various compartments and carefully keep your items in it. You need a durable and easy to carry a backpack that can accommodate all your essential items. Basic Tools to Care your Family

You should keep Antiseptic Wipe with you. Sterile gloves are important for a first aid kit.

Make sure to keep triangular Bandages with you.

The Crepe Bandages are also important. Safety pins will help you to secure your tents and clothes. These are used in a multipurpose way.

Make sure to have sterile plaster in every size, from small to large.

The water purification chemical or tablets are important.

Keep extra water with you for your initial days to peacefully find a new water stream.

Important Medicines to Keep with You

There are some medications that you should keep in your first aid kit, such as:

Paracetamol

Antacids

Aspirin

Dihydrocodeine

Ibuprofen

Tablets for rehydration

Anti-diarrhea pills

Solution to wash the eyes
Gel and cream to treat burns
Medication to treat insect bites
Sunscreen
Blister and sanitary pads
CPR Mask
Sterile Kits Should Have:
Silk stitch and needle
Strips to close wounds
Dressings with adhesives (all sizes from small to large)
Important tools to Keep with You:
Scissors and knives
Pen, pencil, and paper
String and duct tape
Small Torch
Threads and needles

Moreover, you can keep any special medicine with you that are linked to any chronic health condition. It will be good to become the part of the first aid training program to learn basic first aid skills, such as treatment of wounds, initial treatment of cardiovascular patients and several other basic to advanced skills. These will help you to save the life of your loved ones and other people around you.

Chapter 13: How to Prepare Your Nut and Fruit Orchard

Make sure you know why you need a Fruit and Nut Orchard

Many new or intending homesteaders have a checklist that lists the essential items they need to succeed.

Ask yourself why you would like to grow a fruit and nut orchard, and how it could benefit you in your homesteading journey. Think about what you will gain from this investment and how you can prepare for the work involved in growing an orchard.

After considering all the factors, we made the decision to plant heirloom and hardy figs, cherries, chestnuts, hardy almonds and pawpaw.

Apples were a favorite food of our family from their infancy. My boyfriend, who had four apple trees, gave me the opportunity to enjoy the deliciousness of apple sauce. From a cherry tree outside my childhood home, I made jam every year. It was something we really enjoyed, even though we were sometimes nostalgic.

Making cherry jam and apple sauce is only one aspect of learning how to make cider. This will also be an important factor in selecting the heirloom apples that we will be growing. As we dig deeper into this subject, sit tight.

We love almonds so it was natural that we plant them.

Growing figs has always drawn me to them. The fruit can be used in baking and cooking in many ways. The addition of figs and other fruits to our orchard reduces the carbon footprint of planting in the backyard.

Select a Good Location for Your Orchard

A healthy orchard will thrive if it receives moderate sunlight and has a rich soil.

While sunlight can have its downsides, it is vital in this instance. You can map out the sun's movements daily and observe when it rises or sets. These details are important because they help you to get to know the climate you want to cultivate, and will assist you in planning your orchard. A minimum of six hours of sunlight per day is required for fruit trees in an orchard. Because I live in Wisconsin, I would say seven to eight hours. You should be careful with deciduous trees. Mark the location you want to plant and ensure that it gets sunlight every day.

To get rid of Buckthorn and dead Ash trees that could affect the growth of the berries, we stake the intended orchard area. Because Buckthorn helps to provide nutrients for the soil, South-Eastern Winsconsin has a lot of clay soils. It makes the soil more moist and improves its potential health.

If you are unsure about the soil type of the area you have marked, dig a hole and examine the layers of soil in that region. Use a web soil map after the analysis to see the soil in your area that has been surveyed previously. Mulch and stray can be added to the soil and there is nothing to lose.

The slope's gentleness and mildness should also determine where the truth is located. Trees that have a gentle slope and good soil get moderate drainage. Their feet don't get too wet. For the root health, drainage is crucial.

Also, you want to make sure that you have easy access to the site so you can observe it every day. They chose the spot right behind the farmyard because they could see it from their living room window. The owner can also access it via his back door.

Plan Your Orchard

You can map your plot using software or graph paper. I spent up to a month outside, using a tape measure to determine how much space was available and how many trees could be fit in that space.

Make sure you do your research about the height and width of each tree so that you can place them appropriately. This is vital as you want all trees to receive enough sunlight. My trees average between 18-20' in height and range from 15-20 to 20' in spread. Your property should have the tallest tree on the north and the shortest trees to the south. This will allow each tree to receive the 6+ hours of sunlight it needs.

Once you have cleared your land, you can then mark it.

Certain fruits you can easily plant in your garden

Homesteading is a goal that everyone has. Some people enjoy the idea of growing their own food for its old-fashioned, friendly nature. Some people are looking to build long-term dependency or protect themselves against natural disasters and crises. The rest will help you save money at the grocery store. It is also a great way to give back. It is a great idea to grow the entire thing I eat, even though vegetables and eggs are easy to produce.

Certain fruits can thrive in many climates and are easy to grow with moderately low skill. This list of ten fruits is worth considering, regardless of whether you're a novice gardener or an experienced one.

Strawberries

Our top pick for the easiest fruit to grow is Strawberries. Because they can be planted in any container, whether it is a floppy basket, ground or bowl, they are very adaptable. They germinate quicker in well-drained soil and with lots of sunlight. Remove any runners as your strawberries grow. This will increase fresh germination and produce more fruit. High beds are a good choice for strawberries. This helps to fight weeds and maintain the soil's quality and shape.

Watermelon

Watermelon plants are so fun to grow, especially for children who love water plants. Watermelon can be too dry so they need to be water-appreciating. They are also delicious and nourishing.

Blueberries

Blueberries thrive in acidic soils and produce nutritious berries towards the end of the summer. These berries can be grown in the ground, or in bowls. We recommend planting them in the ground as a feature of a remodel, because they will grow beautiful, sweet-smelling flowers in spring.

Only choose blueberry plants that can self-pollinate when you are choosing your garden. You will need to plant more than one plant in order to harvest the fruit. This can make it difficult to manage.

Raspberries

Raspberry, affectionately known as homestead classic, germinates well in places that were previously withered by fire. This fruit is a good opportunity to grow in acidic soils. There are both summer- and fall-fruiting varieties. They need good drainage and plenty of sunlight. They can thrive in the shade, depending on which variety they are given.

This is important: After harvesting raspberries, remove any branches that produced fruit. Other branches will still be available for next year's production and the plant won't need to make extra effort to fix them.

Apples

People claim they have great success planting apples into containers and pots, but I prefer to plant them directly in the ground. They love full sun and well-drained soils. To increase growth, make sure they are trimmed each winter.

Keep in mind the possibility that your apple trees might not produce the same kind of apples as you're used to. Wild apples can be eaten safely, as they have thicker skins and a bitter flavor.

They can be used for baking and fed to livestock.

Pears

Pears look beautiful and add a sweetness to desserts and dinners. Pears can be grown against a wall/lattice, or as dwarfing rootstock bushes.

It is best to have more than one tree, even if one tree is self-sufficient. This will ensure that you are safe and produce a lot of fruit. They are also delicious when made into syrup.

Plums

Plum trees are one of the easiest to grow, but many homesteaders overlook them. Plum trees are self-fertile (don't require pollination), and they produce a lot of fruit from mid to late summer.

When growing plum trees, ensure that they are at least 2 inches apart. It is also important to thin the fruit in order to ensure that it develops properly and produces a good crop next year.

Place them against a wall to allow them to spread outwardly.

Figs

Figs are trees that are so fond of the sun and can add a Mediterranean touch to any dish. They are great for side dishes and salads because of their edible flavor. They can also be dried for future use and taste great on their own.

It is better to keep figs indoors during winter because they won't be able to survive without protection. Make sure that the plant has all of its nutritional requirements met, including compost and other supplements.

Peaches

China is the source of the USA's first peach tree, which can thrive in USDA zones 5 through 8. Peaches prefer to be in warmer climates. They do well in moderate temperatures.

If you live in extreme weather, it is best to choose dwarf varieties to grow in containers and pots. They will eventually outgrow the pots. To conserve moisture, the plants should be kept well hydrated in their pots using vermiculite or peat moss.

Plan and plant your vegetables and herbs

Healthy and balanced diets are those that include a variety of nutrients. Although it may seem impossible to find this in our daily lives, it may not be impossible if you are reliant on the quality of what you make.

A reliable supply of vitamins, minerals and attractive vegetables can be the solution to all your problems. You can also create a variety of invasive plants and get a guide for survival.

In Four Easy Steps, How to Plant a Garden

Decide what you want to plant

This is the fun part. Start by listing all the recipes that you frequently create. You should include vegetables and herbs that you use often. This will help you decide not only what to plant but also how much.

Do not forget to note any other foods that your family likes, even if they aren't being used in your current meal preparation. A garden can be a great way to broaden your culinary horizons.

This is a good time to get your children interested in farming. If they are too young or unable to come up with ideas, you can ask them for suggestions. Children of all ages love sunflowers, decorative gourds and pumpkins for their beauty and delicious seeds. Quick-growing plants, like lettuce and beans are great choices for young people because they produce quick results.

Once you have a list of plants that you want to grow, you can start collecting purchase order catalogs. You can also search online or visit your local garden center to find seeds and transplants. These resources will help you learn a lot about what plants grow well in your area.

Choose a location for your garden

Like real estate, the key to a successful garden is location, location and location. There are certain things that you will have to do if you want your plants to flourish.

1. Sunshine: Choose a sunny spot with at least 6 hours of direct sunlight per day.

2. Water: Make sure you have easy access to water at the place you choose. Sometimes Mother Nature will force you to water your plants. In these cases, ensure that you have a reliable supply of water within arm's reach.

3. Accessibility: Gardeners love to be cared for, so place your garden in an area that is easy to reach with a wheel barrow. It will be tempting to abandon it if it is too far from your house or garden shed where you keep your tools, or in an area that is difficult to reach with a wheelbarrow. Plant your garden in the best spot for sun exposure.

4. Perfect Drainage: This is a difficult one to achieve, especially if you live in an area with clay or dense soil. You may want to plant to collect standing water if you find the realm. To protect your plants from being too wet, you might also wish to make sure your beds are well-made.

Create Your Garden Beds

After you've decided where you want your garden to be, it may be necessary to place the individual beds. Be aware of how the sun moves through the day. If taller plants are used or trellises are used, they can create shadows that cause damage. Many senior faculty gardeners recommend the traditional method of removing layers of sod to make individual beds. Then, cultivate and amend the soil below before you plant your vegetables. This method is effective, but you don't have to do it so hard. Instead of digging into your garden to make them, you can use Lasagna Gardening Methodology. This method works well for both raised garden beds and directly on the ground. Start by adding a thick stack newspaper or flattened cardboard to the top of your ground. Next, you will add layers of topsoil and peat.

These beds can be prepared months in advance or just before planting. The layers can be merged together to create a beautiful, well-made soil for your plants.

Fast-Growing Vegetables to Use in Your Homestead

* Spinach

Spinach is a delicious and nutritious plant that can be harvested. Cool climates are best for spinach. To maximize your space, plant two spinach plants in succession.

Although spinach is not recommended for hot weather, it can be grown in spring and early summer.

When to plant: The first crop should be planted approximately four weeks before the last day of your last expected day. The second harvest should be planted between 6-8 weeks after your last day of freezing.

Harvest Days: The leaves can be harvested within 20 days once they are the right size. Take out the outer leaves first, and harvest for a longer time.

* Kale

It's delicious and easy to grow. It can grow to 20 degrees Fahrenheit in cool climates, just like other vegetables with kale leaves. It is usually good in cold weather. Ideal are a fall and spring crop. Kale can be grown in winter at USDA locations 7-9.

When to plant: A spring harvest should be planted approximately four weeks before the last frost date. A second crop can then be planted in late summer, or early fall.

Harvest Days: The leaves are fully ripe after 60 days. However, small leaves can still be harvested once they reach the size of your fingers. If you want to harvest the plant while it is still ripe, make sure you have at least four leaves.

* Arugula

It has a bold, green flavor. Arugula, another leafy plant that grows quickly, can be harvested carefully to maximize its effects. This is the end of the growing season. If you notice flowers on the plant, this means that the plant has finished its growth cycle.

When to Plant: Start planting a few weeks before last frost and the second crop should be in the fall.

Harvest Days: 20 days young leaves, 40 days ripening

* Radish

The seedling is one of the easiest plants to grow. It comes in both spring and winter varieties. Spring varieties grow much faster than winter. To check their growth, pull on the leaves or press the soil to see if bulbs are formed. They produce incredible quantities. They produce bigger plant sizes, but they are not different nutrients.

When to plant: Seeds should be planted approximately four weeks before the last frost.

Harvest Days: Spring varieties take 20-30 days, winter varieties can take up to 60 days.

* Lettuce

It is a delicious side dish to most foods. Lettuce can be grown in cold climates and will respond well to the same harvesting methods as other leafy vegetables. For best results, plant spring and fall crops.

When to plant: Spring crops should be planted approximately four weeks before last frost day. Spray the plants four weeks prior to the first day of freezing.

Harvest Days: The leaves take 40 days to fully ripen. However, the leaves can still be harvested at any stage of the growth.

* Beans

Beans can be grown in a variety of ways, and they are easy to store in nutritious areas. Beans are nutritious and can be eaten raw or dried quickly. Some beans grow easily without support (bush beans), while others require support to produce delicious pole beans.

When to plant beans: Beans should be planted when the soil remains warm.

Harvest Days: Most beans mature in 60 days. However, some beans can take up 100 days.

* Snap Peas

Delicious, nutritious, high-quality, and fast-growing. What more can you want? There are many types of peas, but snap peas are the most popular. You can eat them as soon as you harvest them. The pod and everything are ready for consumption as soon as possible. The more pods you select, the more productive your plant will be.

When to plant: A few days before the final suspension. Cold can cause peas to become sensitive.

Harvest Days: 40-60 days. It is important to pick more peas to get a good yield.

* Green Onions

Green onions have many nutritional benefits, but their primary purpose is to add flavor and color to your diet. A few green onions mixed with soup can make a dish sing. It is also great for accompanying meat dishes. Your imagination is your limit when it comes to cooking.

When to Plant: Onions like warm soil, so wait until your last frost day before you plant.

Harvest Days: It takes approximately 50 days for the poles to reach maturity. The poles can be harvested as soon as they reach about 5" in height. However, this can reduce the growth of the onion bulb.

* Carrots

Because carrots grow far beyond what we can see, their growth is difficult. It is important to plan correctly. You should give carrots a chance to grow in sandy soil. Make sure to add lots of compost to the garden before you start to plant them. To watch their growth, plant lots of carrots.

When to plant: Four weeks before the frost.

Harvest Days: Carrots are ready to harvest when they have ripened for about 60 days.

* Turnip

A great source of fiber, and antioxidants. Turnips are a reliable, easy-to-grow and strong vegetable that can be used in any garden for healthy eating. They can be used as part of potatoes by some people, but they are not my favorite vegetable.

When to plant: In September, with the fall crop. Turnips can be grown in winter in warmer climates (USDA 9-10).

Harvest Days: 30-60 days. Turnip greens may be harvested in 30 days but full maturity takes 60 days.

* Tomatoes

Tomatoes are one of my favourite vegetables, despite the fact that they require a lot of water. To get the best results when growing, harvesting and collecting seeds for next season, choose heirloom tomatoes. Heirloom tomatoes are delicious plants that can be easily sown. They also produce endless tomatoes, which can survive until their death from cold. Box Car Willie is my favorite.

When to plant: After the first snowfall in spring. If possible, it is best to plant two to four weeks before the last frost in your house.

Harvest Days: On average, harvest takes 60 days. Harvest days: 60 days on average.

The Homestead should grow great healing herbs

I love to grow medicinal plants and herbs in my garden. Growing food is a passion of mine, but the best thing about growing herbs to make medicinal products is even more satisfying!

Why do you plant healing herbs?

This is the obvious answer: I can make natural remedies for any illness in my family! Growing my own medicine is important for several reasons.

I have chronic health issues that are not being treated by conventional medicine. Natural remedies have allowed me to manage my severe health problems and reduce my symptoms.

-Herbal remedies can be expensive to purchase!

I control the herbs that go into my herbal remedies.

There are many reasons to grow herbs.

* Easier to grow - Most are easy to grow even for those who have a black thumb or gardener.

* Attractive – I love to look out in the garden to see beautiful flowers that are attached to my vegetables.

* Other Plants – Herbs can be grown with non-plants, so there is no need for them to have their own space. But you can, if it works best for your needs. These are the best.

* Pest Control – Many herbs repel pests and attract good bugs.

It is easy to see how it can be used to help you develop your healing remedies. It is easy to get overwhelmed by all the medicinal plants available and how they can be used.

Keep it simple, my advice. Start by identifying a few common healing herbs that you feel will be most beneficial for your family. It's better to take the time to build your home medicine cupboard than do nothing.

Amazing Healing Herbs and their Use

There are many herbal remedies I could add to this list. But these are the ones I use. They are versatile and beautiful, as well as being functional. Every year, each one finds a home in my garden.

* Lavender

You may have seen me before and know I love lavender. It is so sweet and fragrant that I cannot help but touch it as it grows. It attracts pollinators and can be easily grown, making it an excellent medicine to new farmers. Lavender is an antiseptic that's warm and powerful.

Here are some ways that lavender can be used

It is a soothing and relaxing experience that can also be comforting for the soul and mind.

Memory improvement

It supports wound healing.

These effects have been observed in me personally. When I smell lavender, I feel calm!

How to use it

The lavender buds and leaves can be added to the carrier oil (coconut or avocado oil, etc.). This can be done by heating the oil and herbs gently for 30 minutes, or by exposing them for a few days to the sunlight. You can store medicinal properties all year long by incorporating oil.

Lavender essential oil or oil is something I love to include in my skincare products, such as face wash or deodorant. You can use lavender at night for any type of product.

Make a coolant. Heat the honey and lavender oil together. Let cool in a small saucepan or tin. This could also be used to hydrate the skin.

* Calendula

Calendula can also be called pot marigold, but it should not be confused with French margold. This remedy blooms with the help of a calendar, which is how it got its name. It's beautiful and practical and one of my favourite options because of its beauty. Calendula offers many benefits.

* Reduce inflammation.
* Supports immune system.
* Calming Cramps

* Supports skin treatments.

Calendula is used in the treatment of salves, for humans as well as animals and pets.

How to use it:

Calendula can be added to the management oil and then to the beehive section. This will make it a homemade herbal remedy. Instead of using antiseptic oils, cut and spread the calendula.

Calendula tea can be a simple way to make a big impact. This post from The Nerdy Farm Wife explains 14 uses for calendula tea.

Calendula leaves make a wonderful addition to salads. These leaves will brighten up any vegetable plate!

* Chamomile

Chamomile can be enjoyed as a lovely and easy-growing plant. This mild, but delicious-tasting tea is what I love to include in my daily herbal tea routine.

It has numerous medicinal properties. Chamomile has been used for centuries by traditional medicine practitioners. Science is now following suit.

Chamomile can be used to:
Encourage rest and sleep
Healthy blood sugar
Calm a fussy baby
Apply a soothing cream to the skin if it is irritated due to eczema
Chamomile, a mild herb, is great for creating calm and balance in stressful modern lives.
How to use it:
* Chamomile is a wonderful vegetable plant that can be used to make tea or for drinking. The plant's glittering flower heads can be easily removed and dried on the screen.

To make an herbal salve, chamomile can be added to carrier oil. This salve will soothe itchy skin.

Chamomile extract can also be used to cleanse hair. Chamomile tea infusion can be used to cleanse your hair and reduce scalp irritation. It will also naturally lighten the hair's color.

Chamomile extract can be used to reduce redness, soothe skin irritations (anti-inflammatory), and reduce blemishes.

* Sage

I love to reach down and rub the rough-textured green leaves of my sage (Salvia Officinalis), between my fingers. Many herbs lose strength as the leaves get larger over the course of the season. Sage is a different case. The more leaves you have, the better the taste.

Sage has been praised for its healing properties for years. Its scent clears my mind and cleanses it. But, sage also has other healing properties.

* Helps to fight cold and flu.
* Reduces pain and swelling
* Aids in fighting infections

Sage is an excellent cooking ingredient, but it's also a powerful medicinal remedy. I have used it in herbal medicine many times.

How to use it:

* Sage is an excellent herb to use in the kitchen during winter and fall. It aids in digestion of rich and heavy grains during the cold season.

It can also be used as a mouthwash. It can be used twice daily to prevent gum irritation and canker sores.

* The sage is often added to deodorants to aid in sweat elimination because it dries.

* Aloe Vera

Growing Aloe vera is easy and fun. Aloe vera grows well in sunny areas, but my experience has shown that it does best when there is no direct sunlight.

Aloe is a desert plant so it doesn't need water. Although aloe is often associated with sunburn, it can be used for many other purposes.

* Moisturise the skin
* To soften the skin
* Treats insect bites, eczema, rash, and burns
* Supports heart health

Aloe vera can be used in many ways.

How to use it:

* Take the leaf from the base of your plant and slice it. Use a spoon to remove the gel from the leaf's center. You can store the leaf in the refrigerator for up to 4 weeks in a glass jar.

This gel can be used to treat any kind of burn, cut, or wipe.

* You can eat it, but you should not ingest bottled aloe vera. Aloe vera softens both the inside and the skin in the same way.

Peppermint

One puff of peppermint oil will give you the energy to water your garden and weed it. Although it won't give you all the energy that you need, it will definitely help you get ahead.

Peppermint wants to overtake your garden so be sure to give it plenty of space when you plant directly into the ground. This herb is known for its digestive health. It can also be used to relax migraines and headaches.

How to use it:

To aid digestion, drink peppermint tea following a heavy meal.

Peppermint oil is great for energy and can be used in the shower to get you through the day. Peppermint oil can be added to shampoo and conditioner. This oil is good for your scalp and can promote hair growth.

* Fresh peppermint leaves can be used to make a tincture. These tinctures can be used immediately to receive the full healing power of the drug. Tinctures can also be easily taken under the tongue and kept well.

* In the summer, add peppermint leaves to your cold or lemon tea. This is a great way for you to cool off inside

* Thyme

Thyme is a wonderful plant that can be used for both medicinal and cooking purposes. Thyme is a sun-loving, fast-growing plant that has been used for many years to increase immunity. When added to chicken or turkey dishes, the small leaves give off a strong flavor.

-Helps to support the body's fight against flu and cold

-Supporting healthy cell growth

Thyme can also be used in cooking if you have it in your kitchen or garden.

How to use it:

Thyme can be added to honey to make it more effective. Honey is enough to make flu and cold symptoms bearable. However, adding thyme to honey increases its potency. Honey can soothe a sore throat or dry cough. Thyme's immune-boosting properties will help your body fight off any illness caused by bugs. You can add thyme honey as a tea flavor or take a teaspoon throughout the day if you feel sick.

* Fresh or dried thyme can be used in soups and dishes. This flavor combination is delicious and fresh! The antioxidant benefits of thyme will be beneficial to the entire family, not just for dinner.

* Garlic

Garlic is a key ingredient in this list of herbs. Garlic can be grown easily, provided you have enough sunlight and the right drainage. This versatile plant has been a great help in my family's fight against the flu and cold. Garlic scapes can also be used to give a garden a formal appearance and to make a pesto for pasta dishes.

* Prevents swelling
* Promotes healthy heart function
* Aids in wound healing
* Increases cell turnover

Garlic is one my favourite spices that I can add to my dishes for aroma and is one of the most simple home remedies you can make.

How to use it:

* A quick way to use garlic is by cutting a clove in half, and then rubbing it onto your skin. This promotes healing.

To nourish your body, eat raw garlic when you are ill.

* Make fire cider – A traditional mix that includes garlic and other spicy herbs. This can be used as a support remedy for the flu and cold.

*Ginger

Ginger is an important ingredient in your kitchen (and your food). Our home. Ginger's many health benefits have been well-known throughout the herbal community. It is well-suited for use in cold and flu conditions.

Ginger is a native of Asia and can be hardy in North America. If you live in a cool area, the ginger plant will need to be brought inside. Ginger powder:

* Help relieve Nausea.

* To aid in sore muscle recovery and overused muscles.
* Menstrual cramps can be relieved.

Ginger is simple to prepare and delicious!
How to use it:

* When I have a sore throat, or a stuffy nose, I prefer to boil fresh ginger root pieces on the stove. For an immune-boosting, warm drink, add honey and crushed lemon juice.
* A hot bath with Epsom Salt is another way to use ginger to relax tired muscles and detoxify your body.

Ginger naturally has a warm flavour and scent. If you don't want to feel cold on winter nights, add it to soups or curries. Ginger in cauliflower rice with turmeric is also a favorite of mine.

* Rosemary

Rosemary's powerful scent is reflected in its light, unforgettable fragrance. Rosemary is very similar to lavender, with its long, thin stalk. Their aromas are quite different, but they smell almost the same. Rosemary is perhaps best-known for its ability to improve memory. However, it has many healing benefits beyond just the brain.

* It relieves your cough.
* Supports the nervous systems.
* Enhances cognition.

Rosemary is also rich in vitamins, minerals and antioxidants which makes it an excellent addition to any kitchen.

How to use it:

* Rosemary oil can be mixed with oil to make a healing salve to treat minor cuts and bruises.

In shampoos and conditioners, pepper mint is often paired with rosemary. This combination smells great and can help improve hair thickness and growth.

* Add rosemary to your favorite chicken dish. You can also make a fragrant oil for cooking with rosemary sprigs.

Chapter 14: Ways To Become An Urban Homesteader

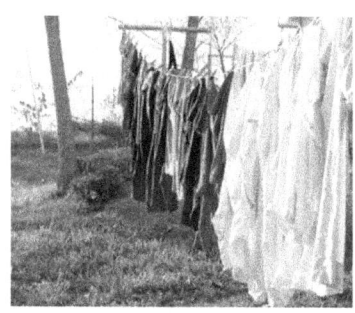

Here are some of the ways to embrace the urban homesteading lifestyle and mentality of eco-friendliness, slow living, and self-sufficiency.

Hang your clothes. Yes, we are used to throwing our clothes in the dryer right after they are washed, but it is much more eco-friendly to hang them. Hanging them is not much of a chore. It is easy even without a clothesline. Just use a drying rack or clothing rack and hangers. You get to dry your clothes without consuming electricity or using and eventually throwing away drying sheets.

Reduce the toxins in the air by taking care of houseplants. Trees are extremely helpful to filter out the air and remove toxins. While it might be impossible to take care of large trees inside your home, you can still reduce those nasty toxins by taking care of some houseplants. If this is your first time gardening, do not lose hope if your plants die on your first try. Giving it another whirl will let you learn how to properly take care of them.

Use organic, chemical-free cleaners. Some people have the impression that urban homesteaders are slobs and dirty. Do not allow yourself to be given that impression by still maintaining the cleanliness and freshness of your home. If you are not cleaning because you do not want to use chemicals, well, that is just an excuse. Because there are a lot of chemical-free and non-toxic cleaners that you can buy or even make to effectively clean your home and your garden. One cost-effective organic all-purpose cleaner is the white vinegar spray. Just simply purchase a spray bottle and white vinegar. Fill ½ of the bottle with white vinegar and ½ with water. Spray the surfaces that you want to clean and wipe them down with an old rag or t-shirt. To keep your backyard clean, just sweep or rake everyday.

Grow your own food. If you have a space for a garden, plan out how to companion garden your plants. Choose the plants that you want to grow and eat, and then choose the plants that will encourage their growth and help protect them from pests and insects. If you do not have enough space outside, the good news is, you can still grow your food in pots and indoors. Nothing is more rewarding than harvesting and eating fruits and vegetables that you planted and grew yourself. Growing your own food will give you satisfaction and help the environment.

Walk or ride public transportation. One of the best assets of living in the city is the accessibility. Cities usually have a lot of public buses and subway train systems, which you can ride instead of bringing your own car. If the place you are going to is just a block or 2 away, try walking. Besides, walking is better for your health too.

Instead of buying pets, adopt. If you are looking for a pet, instead of looking for one in pet stores, look for it in your local shelters. You are helping and basically giving an animal a family and a home.

Learn how to compost. Instead of immediately throwing out the trash, try to save the things that can be used for compost. Garbage can be transformed into rich soil that can be extremely helpful and beneficial to your plants. While you might not want to get your hands dirty at first, the process is actually very simple. So save those banana peels and even the manure of your backyard animals for composting.

Buy from thrift shops or garage sales. Urban homesteading encourages you to think before buying or spending. If there is really a need for you to buy, let's say a clothing rack for your clothes to hang from, instead of going directly to the mall, look for one in thrift shops or garage sales. A lot of people throw out stuff in good condition and you will be able to get it at a fraction of the price. Buying used stuff is always an eco-friendly way to shop and also a really great way to save money.

Share. This is very easy to do if you know your neighbors and the other people in your community. Instead of having your own lawn mowers, tools, or snow blowers, why not share instead? You can always take and borrow from one another. If you do not know your neighbors, talk to them and offer yours. In this way, when they have something that you need to borrow, you can just ask to borrow it and not have to buy one that you will rarely use anyway.

Buy local items. Support the local industry and buy your necessities from the farmer's market. The reason why buying local items is better for the environment is because you are not buying an imported item that has to use tons of fuel, causing air or water pollution just to be shipped. Visit your local farmer's market, fairs, and the local shops around your community.

Resist the desire to buy stuff. It is very easy for people to get sucked into the consumeristic world we are in now. We are always slapped with advertising schemes and marketing strategies, that, let's admit, can be very convincing. These schemes and strategies make us believe that we need what they are selling even if we do not. If we get tempted to what they are pitching, we not only add more clutter to our lives, but we are also damaging the environment because it is something that sooner or later, we'll realize we do not need and just simply throw it out.

Choose experiences over material possessions. One very effective way to reduce your consumption of the earth's limited resources is to learn how to value experiences more than material possessions. For example, instead of buying yourself a new gift for your birthday, why not go on a trip to a different country instead? This is an experience that you will never forget and replace. You get to see new sights, meet new people, and learn a different culture. While this may be a birthday gift for yourself that does not come in a fancy packaging, it is a gift that will surely never end up in your trash or in your next garage sale.

Use alternative sources of energy. Urban homesteading can be attained one step at a time, but at some point, you will need to find some alternative sources of energy to fully embrace an eco-friendly lifestyle. Before you purchase some of these eco-friendly devices though, make sure that you research and study them first to make sure that you are buying the ones that really suit what you need. There are different alternative sources of energy such as solar, wind, and geothermal. These devices, although expensive, are becoming more and more popular because they become really cost-effective in the long run.

Collect rainwater. Collecting rainwater can either be complicated or simple. If you really want to replace the water that you usually use with rainwater, you might need to purchase expensive setups and have them installed in your home. Just like alternative sources of energy, although expensive, these setups can become extremely helpful and cost-effective in the long run. If you do not want to shell out your money on expensive water systems, you can simply place a barrel in your yard and wait till the rain falls. The water that you collect can be used to water your garden, clean your garage, wash your car, wash the dishes, and even flush toilets.

Grow fruit trees. If you want to get into the habit of growing and eating your own food, but cannot fully commit to a whole lot of upkeep right away, a good idea is to start by planting a few fruit trees. These fruit trees can be planted right in your backyard or in containers that can be placed inside your home. These trees need to be fully settled and established before they start producing fruit, but fortunately, they are very easy to maintain. You can grow lemons, oranges, apricots, cherries, avocados, pomegranates, and even figs. There are a lot of fruit trees to choose from, however, you will need to consider how much light your home gets and how often you can tend to your plants before you finally pick which ones to grow.

<small>Learn to compost.</small> Composting is extremely helpful and cost-effective. Set aside all the banana peels, eggshells, grass clippings, and coffee grounds. Some of the things and foods that you usually throw in the trash can actually be a good source of free, rich, and healthy soil that can help nurture and encourage the growth of your plants. Composting is one of the most basic components that you need to learn when you want to grow your own food. When you turn waste into something useful, you not only get to save, but you also reduce the trash, which helps the environment.

<small>Recycle creatively.</small> There are so many things and ways that you can recycle. Egg shells, egg cartons, and even toilet paper rolls can be used in place of pots to grow small plants in, old t-shirts can be cut up and used as rags, cardboard boxes can be used to straighten your plants or as a weed barrier, old plastic bottles, jars, and even glass bottles can be used to store random things and cereal boxes can be turned

inside out so they can be used as boxes. Every time you want to throw something out, think of other things you can use it for. If something is broken, try to fix it first before replacing it with a new one.

Bake your own bread. Baking your own bread is actually easy and will not take you one whole day. However, you might need to try a few different recipes before you finally find the one that you like. When you make your own bread, you do not have to add in preservatives or chemicals to prolong its shelf life, because you can make just the right amount that you can consume. Aside from that, your bread will always be fresh.

Take care of backyard chickens. Backyard chickens are very easy to take care of and you do not need a large garden to take care of them. You just have to give them a chicken coop and enough space for them to roam around. Before you decide to buy chickens, you have to drop by your local municipality first to learn about the laws and city rules.

Reduce your consumption of electricity. Consciously make an effort to reduce your use of electricity throughout your day. Unplug any gadget or appliance that you are not using, if you need to buy new ones, choose Energy Star, replace your light-bulbs with energy-efficient ones, lower your thermostat, especially during colder seasons or higher during warmer seasons, if it's hot, instead of turning on the air conditioning unit, open your windows to let the breeze in, if it's cold, open your blinds or window shades to let the warmth of the sun in, turn off the lights when not in use, hang your clothes instead of putting them in the dryer, wash only when you have a full load, etc.

Tips for urban homesteading

Unclutter. When you decide that you want to be an urban homesteader, the first step that you should do is to unclutter your life. We live in a world with so much unnecessary excess—whether it's material possessions, emotional baggage, or life stresses. Find a way to fully appreciate the simpler things in life. Spend more time with family and friends, nurture your relationships, develop hobbies, experience new places, things, events, cultures, etc. instead of working 24/7 so you can pay off your debt because of things that you cannot not only afford, but do not need as well.

Make things yourself. You have to realize that you can make almost everything that you need to survive, yourself. You can make your own shampoo, soap, and lotion that are free from any chemicals that can harm your health. You can even make your own bread without having to add preservatives. You can plant your own fruits and vegetables so you will always have fresh and organic food to munch on. Being able to successfully make things yourself is extremely rewarding and brings you a different kind of satisfaction. Making things yourself will bring you peace of mind, save you money, and protect your health.

Take care of small animals. Keeping livestock is really helpful. You can raise chickens or even rabbits, if you want your animals to be quiet. Their manure can be used as compost, which enables you to save money on fertilizers.

Utilize the sun. Invest in a solar oven. This is one great way to save on your energy bill and will do a good job at cooking your meals.

Be realistic. You do not have to do everything all at once. You can practice urban homesteading one step at a time.

Chapter 15: How To Create An Amazing Homestead Garden

Maybe I'm wrong, but I feel like there is a huge difference between a farm garden and a homestead garden. Farming is so honest and gritty. Farming is about getting dirty, working hard, staying focused and above all else, getting stuff done. And I feel the typical farm garden reflects that utilitarian sentiment.

Farm gardens are wildly productive, abundant and ordered,crops are often planted in rows, evenly spaced and straightforward. There is no time to explore or to just be with the plants, there is no time to let the garden determine your next meal. You tromp focused down the row, stop at the expected aisle and harvest just what is needed, taking time only to weed a little and then turn on your boot heels and head back the way you came.

Homesteading, on the other hand, is less about energy in versus calories out and more about place-making. While productivity is equally important in a homestead garden, there seems to be something different about a homestead garden, something that is hard to define, it's almost curious.

This type of gardening draws you in, invites you to stay and quietly welcomes you to become part of it, to touch, smell and taste its wares. To harvest what you see and to search out what you cannot, more like a leisurely treasure hunt than a task that needs doing.

So, what sets this type of garden apart from other forms of gardening, why is it so much more magical than a common production garden? And how do you create a garden like this for yourself? All you have to do is follow these 3 simple rules and you will have the homestead garden of your dreams.

Design

Integrate

Adapt

A gorgeous homestead garden is well designed, complexly integrated and adapts with the changing seasons. A homestead garden is more than a place to grow food, it is an extension of the home and is designed to serve the needs of the gardener and their family.

As a homestead gardener myself, this is where the flavours of my kitchen are defined, where my herbal medicine is harvested and where I go to first to seek nourishment for myself and my family. I am in my homestead garden every day, it is truly a part of my home and as such, I treat it with respect and gratitude.

How to Create an Amazing Homestead Garden - The Hip Homestead

Design

Where to begin? Always Start with a Great Design:

Design is essential for establishing a new garden or even for adapting an old one. Stay focused on how you want your garden to feel, follow the tips below and before you know it you will have a homestead garden worth showing off.

Customize your Homestead Garden

Design with yourself in mind, create a wish list of all of the elements you want in your homestead garden. List the foods you and your family eat most often, the flowers that you love, even your favourite colours and include them in your plan. Doing so will help you establish your must have features and help you create a shopping list when it comes time to pull it all together.

Express your Design Style

Look online for inspiration, if your aesthetic is wild and free then design for that, making sure to stand firm on a few key design rules:

1: tallest items like fruit trees to the back

2: low border plants like strawberry or daylily to the front

3: foot traffic friendly plantings like thyme and sedums on the edges or along the paths

After that, go wild! Design in winding paths that lead to hidden treasures like a rhubarb patch or apple tree.

Create woven willow structures that act as both plant supports and art into your garden, remember this is your space there are no wrong answers.

Use plants that hold their structure and keep spaces and paths clearly defined. To incorporate edibles into your formal homestead garden consider substituting traditional plant species for edible options, for example instead of a boxwood try a blueberry hedge.

When selecting lettuce varieties, opt for colour blocked rows of head lettuce to line your paths. By keeping to plants that hold their shape and colour you will have better luck predicting their final size and shape, resulting in a more formal looking homestead garden.

Keep it Close to Your Home and Easy to Access

Set your garden up for success by keeping it close to your main traffic areas, nothing deteriorates a garden faster than neglect. Place your garden close to the house and in a sunny area that is easy to access.

Design adequate paths and access throughout your homestead garden as well. I prefer my paths to be around 3 feet wide and I always line them with mulch, gravel or grass to help differentiate the paths from the planting beds.

Design in Social Spaces

Homesteaders live where they work and take pride in their homes. Which is why it's nice to design in a bit of peacemaking in your beautiful homestead garden. A spot to sit and read a book or enjoy tea with a friend.

A few things to consider when designing a social space in your homestead garden include the size of the social area, sun exposure, and guest interaction.

How you use the space will help define its size. If you want it large enough to fit the whole family be sure to plan room for dining and seating for everyone. Will your space be used as a place to have a cup of tea with a friend? or just big enough for a lounge chair or two?

Consider designing for shade and sun exposure. Do you want a space to hide from the heat of the day or bask in the sun while sipping a cool herbal ice tea? Design for your needs and lifestyle to get a truly custom garden.

Include elements that entice the senses and evoke interaction between the guests and the garden. Flowers like evening scented stock, lavender, and sweet pea all smell amazing. Wind chimes, birdbaths and garden art all create visual interest in the garden, all of which add to the experience of the garden and encourage your guests to return. Think of ways you can stimulate the senses in your homestead garden.

Ask yourself questions like these early on in the design process to avoid major changes later on. While the design might seem like an easy step to skip, please don't overlook it. A well-designed homestead garden is customized to meet your specific needs, expresses your personal style and is easy to access and maintain, making it an enjoyable space to explore and be a part of; which is what a homestead garden is all about.

Integrate

Use Integration to Create a Gorgeous Garden

Integration is the practice of mixing plant species that are normally segregated, by stacking your crops you can create higher yields in a smaller space. Secondary crops like nasturtium and pumpkin can be set to ramble throughout a home orchard, making use of the lower growing area, attracting bees and creating shade to retain moisture on the orchard floor, integration can be not only productive but incredibly beautiful.

Integration is what defines the homestead garden, herbs and veggies grow under fruit trees, flowers and medicinal herbs grow together and are harvested for use in the home.

An integrated garden is incredibly productive and mimics a natural ecosystem. Designing this way may be a new style of gardening for you but trust me, it's not only productive but beautiful as well, just be sure to include the following 4 elements:

culinary herbs
medicinal herbs
annual vegetables
perennial crops

1: Culinary Herbs

Integrating culinary herbs into your homestead garden is essential if you are planning on gardening with organic practices. Culinary herbs bring in pollinators and confuse pests they also serve as great companions to your other plants.

If you cook often, culinary herbs can quickly rack up your grocery bill, which is crazy because they are so easy to grow. While some are annuals and need to be reseeded each year, many culinary herbs are perennial and can be harvested year after year.

Culinary herbs serve so many uses and are essential in any homestead garden. Fresh spring herbs can easily be harvested with nothing more than a pair of kitchen scissors, dried indoors and stored for use all season long.

Culinary herbs to include in your homestead garden:

Thyme, oregano, cilantro, chive, basil, rosemary, and dill.

2: Medicinal Herbs

Integrating medicinal herbs into a homestead garden is a great way to benefit both you and your garden. Medicinal herbs can be used in the garden as organic pesticides for healthy plants, mulch plants healthy soils and as fodder crops for healthy chickens and livestock if you have them.

The effectiveness of herbal medicine is gaining validation through the medical community and is beginning to be seen as an acceptable alternative to pharmaceuticals for the treatment of minor illness. This is good news for the urban or rural homesteader because homesteaders are tough cookies and won't often bend to treatable upsets. Instead of taking the day off if a tummy ache strikes,they will head out to the homestead garden, brew a pot of mint and fennel tea and then get back to work.

Medicinal herbs like mint, chamomile and dill are generally safe for consumption, but you should consult your physician and do a little reading on exactly how and why before taking anything as a solution to any ailment, doing so will help you avoid side effects or unintended results. And always ask your doctor before taking herbs when pregnant or nursing. Safety first, as always!

Medicinal herbs come in countless forms but are often flowering plants that are not only useful but beautiful as well. The structured silver beauty of a mature lavender plant, the colour explosion of bee balm flowers or the mob of yellow and orange blooms that come with calendula plants are all gorgeous and absolutely worth incorporating into any medicinal homestead garden. Be sure to integrate medicinals into your homestead garden and grow your own "Farmacy".

Medicinal herbs to include in your Homestead garden:

Plantain for bee stings, mint for stomach upset, cilantro to prevent gas, garlic to boost the immune system and lavender for relaxation.

3: Annual Veggies

Growing your own food is rewarding and healthy and as such annual vegetables are essential for any homestead. All too often we segregate our vegetable garden, casting it off to the back yard like an afterthought, just another way to 'deal' with the unsightly corner of the yard.

I feel our food deserves more respect than that, instead, our veggies should hold a place of honour in our yards; the brightest spot close to our social spaces and our kitchens; it's the least we can do for these darling little plants that live to feed us.

Grow your veggies among your herbs and medicinals to create a self-supporting ecosystem. Peas and beans can be trained to climb fruit trees, nasturtium flowers can ramble among squash plants to increase pollination and self-seeding salad greens like lettuce and ruby mustard work well to fill empty space and out-compete weeds.

Annual Vegetables to include in your homestead garden:

Lettuce and salad greens, scarlet runner beans, squash and pumpkin, garlic and onions.

4: Perennial Food Crops

Be sure to include perennial food crops in your integrated homestead garden. Perennials are so easy to grow and once established can grow on for years without any work from you.

I recently consulted on a historical homestead that was established in 1910, where I found perennial crops that are still going strong today, this included 2 massive walnut trees, a diverse fruit orchard that was way older than I am, and asparagus plants that had self-seeded along the length of the driveway. Both the new owners and I were amazed at the resilience of these perennial food crops.

So clearly, homesteaders know the value of perennial crops, species you plant once and they continue to come back year after year.

What could be better than stepping out into your homestead garden to harvest a bushel of fresh rhubarb and a bowl of fresh strawberries and bringing them straight to the kitchen to create a fresh baked pie that holds all the flavours of spring.

Cultivating an annual vegetable garden can be a lot of work, and needs to be redone year after year which is why integrating perennials into your homestead garden can be a wise and delicious decision.

Perennial crops to include in your Homestead garden:

Nut trees, fruit trees, strawberries, rhubarb, berry bushes, french sorrel, and asparagus.

A well-integrated garden is healthy and productive, herbs, fruit, and veggies are planted densely to out-compete weeds confuse pests. Flowers are included to increase pollination, add beauty and attract beneficial insects.

An integrated homestead garden provides crops, habitat and visual interest through the seasons, and with so much to explore it is also an adventure waiting to be had.

Chapter 16: Homestead in the Home

You don't just have the backyard options for homesteading. There are many things you can do inside, especially in winter when there isn't much outside.

You can make soap, shampoo, toothpaste, cleaners and shampoo all at home with organic ingredients.

Here is a simple home soap recipe for you to try, courtesy of www.diynatural.com:

Coconut oil: 2/3 cup

2/3 cup olive oil

1/3 cup grapeseed oil/sunflower oil

1/4 cup lye

3/4 cup water

You can use essential oils or herbs to create a fragrance of your choice

Newspaper can be used to cover your work area. Wear gloves and protective clothing. You will need to measure your water into the canning jar. Use a spoon to measure the water. Make sure to measure 1/4 cup of lye. Slowly add the lye to the water, stirring constantly. To avoid any fumes, stand back and stir the water. You can let the water clear up and then move on to the next step.

Add your oils to a pint jar. You should make one pint. Place the oil in a microwave oven for around a minute. Your oils should be at least 120 degrees. The temperature of your lye should be at 120deg. Let both cool down between 95deg to 105deg. This is crucial for soap making. It will not come together as quickly and will be crumbly and coarse.

Once both oils and lye are at the correct temperature, add the oils to a bowl. Slowly add the oil and stir until everything is well combined. Mix by hand for 5 minutes. It is important that the lye comes in contact with the soap as little as possible. You can continue stirring for about five minutes or use an immersion blender. The soap mixture will become lighter in color and thicken. It will look like vanilla pudding when it reaches "trace".

At this stage, add your essential oils and herbs. Mix well. Mix the ingredients well and pour into molds. Cover with plastic wrap. Wrap the mixture in a towel. Wrap it in a towel to keep any heat from escaping and begin the process of saponification. The process by which the base ingredients are transformed into soap is called saponification.

Check your soap after 24 hours. Allow it to rest for 12-24 hours if it is still warm. Once it's cold and firm, transfer it onto parchment paper or a baking rack. Cut into bars if you used a loaf pan. Let soap cure for about 4 weeks. It is important to flip it once per week to expose the sides to air. This is not necessary if you are using a baking rack. An old potato chip rack was used to make a soap drying rack. I then used cardboard fabric bolts from a fabric shop to slide through the rungs.

Wrap your soap in wax paper once it has fully cured. Handmade soap makes its own glycerin which pulls moisture from the atmosphere. Wrap it to prevent moisture from attracting debris and dust.

Lye is a caustic, and can cause skin or clothing to burn.

One of the most important steps for indoor homesteading is food preservation.Remember all that food you harvested from your Garden of Eden?Now it is time to make it last for the winter, offering fresh, all natural food for your family all year long.

You can freeze or cure meats to preserve them for the winter. Take out what you need for each meal.

You can also make home remedies for your family that are easy to prepare. A quick Google search will reveal many tasks for indoor homesteading.

Chapter 17: Fast Growing Vegetables For A Spring Garden

Do you have this burning desire to have your garden, or are you thinking about getting into the realm of gardening? Planting your food is an excellent step on the road towards attaining self-sufficiency, and the expensive prices of supermarket vegetables are becoming less manageable by the day. Perhaps you're already experienced gardening considering the move to diversify into food, or solely looking for a few new species to hold your interest. Either way, there are some unique species out there, so check below for a few fast-growing spring vegetables to get you started.

i. Spinach

The good news is that you should expect to be harvesting this plant in around 50 days, quite likely less. With luck, you'll be able to harvest the leaves and keep harvesting many times over the long growing season. Not only is this a fast producer, but it's tasty and useful in a variety of meals while providing more than enough leaf to be worth the investment. Consider grasping a plain-leaf specimen, though. They're less prone to hold on to annoying particles of soil, so washing them is a breeze.

ii. Turnips

They're growing unwaveringly more popular. Some fast-growing species like "red milan" will have baby globes available to pull within a few weeks, and from then on will grow rather quickly. Recognize that sometimes turnip's roots can take a surprisingly long time to settle in, but all is not lost. Within 25-30 days most breeds will have produced delicious leaves to be harvested and will likely be available to eat themselves.

iii. Green Onions and Scallions

Shocking enough, these have a catch. They unquestionably are advised as an exceptional spring planting, but not from seed. They take a fair while to grow from seed, but can be gotten ahold of in most garden centers as somewhat grown bunching packs. You could easily get a hundred for a fiver and have edible green onions ready for the chopping board in less than three weeks.

iv. Radishes

They are exceptional for speed alone. Plant them on the first day of March, and you'll be consuming them before April has time to raise its head. 25-30 days is the going rate, for the record. Just don't leave them in much longer, or they start getting springy. They're a good plant to grow with children; push the seeds in between a half and a three-quarter-inch deep, and they'll get to see their work show shortly. Early spring has fewer insects buzzing around, so you should be able to avoid pests as well.

You can now enjoy your garden

These are only a few of the many suitable spring plants, so be sure to check if there's anything more suitable for you out there. Anyway, these are wonderful plants with unique qualities, and investing in them for your spring garden is a step in the right path.

Conclusion

This book fills in as you're above all else direct for homesteading. Homesteading isn't only another sort of planting or some extravagant method of living at present stylish. It is one of the most antiquated strategies rehearsed by a few civic establishments as you have perceived at this point and the nearest approach to living in congruity with nature. It is a lifestyle and a decision you make. I see any change accompanies opposition and doubt particularly when it requires your valuable time and vitality on an everyday premise. In any case, I guarantee you the outcomes are expansive and you will see the astonishing outcomes it brings to you and your family regarding unrivaled nature of wellbeing and consequently life.

Subsequently take this book just as a tenderfoot's guide and keep proceeding with your excursion in to homesteading and natural living with a few different books and web journals. I propose joining your nearby, natural planting clubs to share thoughts and get the support to proceed with this excursion.

www.ingramcontent.com/pod-product-compliance
Lightning Source LLC
Chambersburg PA
CBHW071832080526
44589CB00012B/994